CONTENTS

Introduction

The Breville Smart Fryer is one of the smart appliances for cooking. It looks like a transfer oven and also fries or cooks your food using the transfer method. The hot air revolves around the food placed on the cooking tray. The hot air circulation technology is the same as the transfer method. The heating elements are displayed on the top of the Breville Smart Deep Fryer with a full power fan. The fan helps to circulate the hot air flow evenly in the oven. This will allow you to cook your food quickly and evenly on all sides. Fry your food in much less oil. Take a tablespoon or less than a tablespoon of oil to fry and mash your food. If you want to fry a bowl of potato chips, your oven with the Breville Smart Air Fryer simply fries the potatoes in a tablespoon of oil. Makes your fries crisp on the outside and tender on the inside.

The Breville Smart Fryer is not only used to fry your food, but also to grill your favorite chicken, bake cakes and cookies, and also reheat your frozen foods. It comes with 12 smart cooking modes. These functions are toast, muffin, bake, broil, pizza, cookies, warm, hot, potato, waterproof, dehydrated, and slow cook. It works with an intelligent Element IQ system that finds the cold spot and automatically adjusts the temperature with PID temperature sensing and digital control, giving you even an accurate cooking. Smart ovens automatically adjust the wattage of the heating elements to give you more flexibility when cooking. The smart fryer oven works with double speed transfer technology; With this technique, you can cook your food faster by reducing cooking time by transferring. The smart fryer comes with a display that shows the 12 smart functions, as well as the cooking temperature and time. The smart fryer is also equipped with a built-in oven light, you can turn this light on at any time to see the cooking progress, or it can turn on automatically after the cook cycle is complete.

The Smart Deep Fryer is made from the most durable materials. The oven shell is made of reinforced stainless steel. In the smart oven, quartz is used instead of the metallic element because the quartz responds faster compared to the metallic element. Heat your oven quickly and evenly. The interior of the smart oven is lined with a non-stick coating that makes your daily cleaning process easy. To avoid burns, the oven rack is a self-extracting magnetic shelf. When you open the oven door, the shelves are automatically removed in the middle of the oven.

The Breville Smart Oven Fryer has one of the most flexible cooking appliances that are easy for everyone to handle. It is more than just a toaster that functions as a deep fryer, working pot, slow cooker, and also has the ability to dehydrate food. If air frying alone is not your main goal, this is the right choice for your kitchen. This smart oven works very well to heat food to the right temperature thanks to the transfer technology. It is one of the more expensive toaster ovens in this section. If your priority is more function, good performance, and flexibility, then the *Breville Smart Oven Fryer* is the best choice for your family.

How to Prepare the Smart Oven Before the First Use

It is necessary to empty the smart oven for 20 minutes before the first use to remove any protective substance adhering to the elements. Before testing, first, place your oven in a well-ventilated area and follow the instructions below.

1. First, remove the advertising stickers, multiple covers, or any packing material from the oven.
2. Remove the baking sheet, crumb tray, dehydrator basket or skillet, pizza tray, baking sheet, broil rack, multi-pack rack, and wash in hot water or soapy water with a cloth smooth and pat dry.

3. Take a soft, damp sponge to clean the inside of the oven and dry it well.
4. Place your oven in a well-ventilated area, making sure it is at least 4-6 inches apart on both sides of the oven.
5. Now insert the crumb tray into the oven in place and plug the power cord into an electrical outlet.
6. The oven display will illuminate with an alarm sound, and the function menu will appear, and the default display is in the TOAST menu setting.
7. Now turn the SELECT/CONFIRM dial until the pointer reaches the PIZZA setting.
8. Press the START/STOP button. After pressing this button, the button's backlight glows red, and the digital oven display glows orange with an audible alert.
9. The display shows the heating flashing. After healing is complete, the oven alarms and timer automatically start measurements.
10. After completing the beeping oven cycle warning, turn off the START/STOP backlight, and the oven LCD display will turn white. This will indicate that the oven is ready for its first use.

Chapter 1.Benefits of the Air Fryer

The smart fryer oven comes with several benefits, some of which are as follows:

Healthy and Fatty Foods

The smart fryer oven works with transfer technology. Blow hot air into the cooking pan to cook food quickly and evenly on all sides. When frying your food in a smart fryer, you need a tablespoon or less than a tablespoon of oil. One bowl of fries requires only one tablespoon of oil and makes the fries crisp on the outside and tender on the inside. If you are among the people who like fried food but are worried about extra calories, this kitchen appliance is for you.

Offers 13-in-1 Operation

The Breville smart air fryer oven offers 13 functions in one device. These functions are Toast, Bagel, Bake, Broil, Hot, Pizza, Proof, Air Fry, Reheat, Cookie, Slow Cook, and Dehydrate. These are all smart programs that offer flexible cooking.

Safe to Use

The smart fryer oven cooking appliances is one of the safest compared to a traditional one. While cooking your food, the appliance is closed on all sides; because of this, there is no risk of hot oil splashing on your finger. This is one of the safest frying methods compared to another traditional frying method. A narrow cooking method gives you a splatter-free cooking experience. Smart IQ technology makes the device safer, and there is no possibility of burning food. Smart IQ automatically detects and adjusts the temperature of the item according to the needs of the recipe.

Easy to Clean

The Breville smart fryer oven is made of reinforced stainless steel, and the inner body is coated with non-stick materials. All interior accessories are dishwasher safe. You can wash it in a dishwasher or also wash it with soapy water. The smart fryer cooks your food in much less oil. Less oil means less chaos.

Care and Cleaning

1. Before starting the cleaning process, ensure that the power cord has been unplugged. Allow your oven and accessories to cool to room temperature before beginning the cleaning process.
2. Clean the oven body with a soft, damp cleaning sponge during the cleaning process. When cleaning the glass door, you can use a glass cleaner and a plastic cleaning pad to clean. Do not use metal coatings that can scratch the surface of your oven.
3. The inner body of the oven consists of a non-stick coating. Use a soft, damp sponge to clean the inside of the oven. Apply detergent to a sponge and do not apply it directly to the body of the oven. You can also use a mild spray solution to avoid staining.
4. Before cleaning the components, make sure the oven has cooled down to room temperature and then wipe gently with a soft damp cloth or sponge.
5. Dust the crumb tray with a soft, damp sponge. You can use a non-abrasive liquid cleaner. Apply detergent to a sponge and clean the disc.
6. To clean a frying pan, immerse it in warm soapy water and wash it with the help of a plastic frying pan or a soft sponge.
7. Remember to always dry all accessories thoroughly before placing them in the oven. Put the crumb tray in place before plugging the oven into its socket. Now your oven is ready for the next use.

Chapter 2.How to Use the Breville Smart Air Fryer Oven

Your air fryer oven really couldn't be easier to use. The front opening door allows you access to the racks, which slide in and out to provide easy access to your food before, during, and after cooking.

- Remove the toaster oven from the box.
- Place it on a level surface near a grounded power outlet.
- Plug in the toaster oven
- Remove the trays from the oven. (Before using the oven make sure to thoroughly clean the trays with soap and water.)
- Set the oven to the Pizza function and use the Time button to select 18 minutes. Press the Start button and allow to finish the cooking cycle. Once the cooking cycle has finished, your Breville Mini Smart Oven is ready to use.

Learning the Controls

The great thing about the Breville Mini Smart Oven is that all of the controls are labeled for easy use, so you don't have to bother with confusing dials. Let's take a look at how the Breville Mini Smart Oven works.

Function knob: This knob allows you to select which cooking program you would like. Choose from Toast, Bake, Broil, Roast, Cookies, Reheat, Pizza, and Bagel.

LCD display: Displays the number of pieces of bread, darkness setting, current time, cooking temperature, and amount of time left to cook.

- Temp/Darkness button: Select the temperature or darkness setting for toast.
- Up and Down selection buttons: Use to adjust the time, temperature, and amount of darkness.
- Time/Slices button: Use to adjust the cooking time and number of slices of bread.

A Bit More: Adds a small amount of cooking time. The amount of time varies depending on which cooking program you have chosen.

Start/Cancel button: Starts and stops the cooking process.

- F/C button: Choose Fahrenheit or Celsius.
- Frozen Foods button: Adds extra time to the cooking process in order to defrost frozen foods.

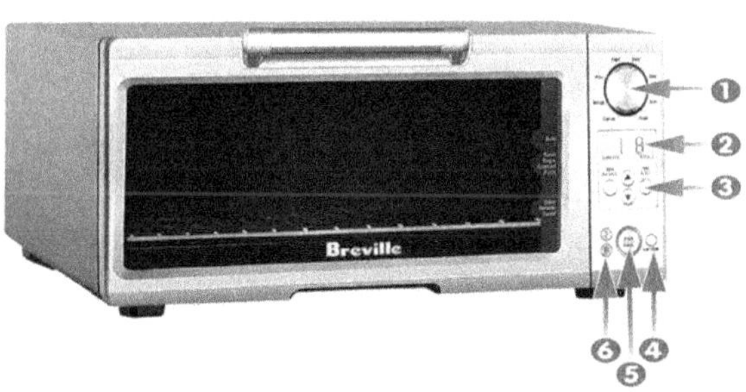

The Cooking Process

The Breville Mini Smart Oven is one of the most advanced toaster ovens on the planet due to its digital controls and Element IQ technology, which regulates the heating elements for optimum results. But perhaps the best feature of the Breville Mini Smart Oven is its ability to cook using convection. Unlike regular baking, convection produces the most even heat possible by circulating the heated air.

It's perfect for many different types of cooking when you want your food to be evenly cooked throughout. It's also a great way to ensure amazing results when baking.

From the moment you choose your cooking program, the Breville Mini Smart Oven begins heating quickly. A great feature of this oven is that it preheats so quickly. And unlike many competing toaster ovens, the Breville Mini Smart Oven allows you to cook up to 450°F, which allows you to cook many foods you would not be able to in other toaster ovens. When the oven finishes cooking, its timer will chime, and it will automatically turn itself off. That's not just a great way to save energy, it's also an important safety feature. After the oven has had a chance to cool, clean it using a damp cloth or sponge to remove any spatter that may have occurred during the cooking process.

Workarounds

We've already explored many of the things your Breville Mini Smart Oven can do, so now let's talk a little about problem solving. When you're cooking in a conventional oven, it is pretty common to line your baking sheets with aluminum foil. It's a great way to keep those baking trays from getting dirty, and that's pretty helpful after your meal. But using aluminum foil in the Breville Mini Smart Oven is not a good idea.

The problem is that using aluminum foil in the Breville Mini Smart Oven can cause the oven to get too hot - sometimes over 500°F - and a toaster oven, unlike your conventional oven, isn't designed to safely work at such a high temperature. To combat this problem and still have a way to line the trays of your toaster oven, try using parchment paper. It will keep food from sticking to the trays, and you can just throw it out after cooking.

You may have noticed that the Breville Mini Smart Oven features a large cooking space inside the oven. As a result, you can cook more efficiently by cooking on several levels at once. While only one cooking rack is included with the oven, you can purchase additional racks. Just make sure to purchase racks in the correct size.

Often, you will see packaged foods with a different temperature recommendation for cooking food in toaster ovens. However, because the Breville Mini Smart Oven cooks almost exactly like a regular oven, it is usually not necessary to use the recommended toaster oven temperature setting. Doing this may actually cause your food to come out overcooked. We suggest that you reduce all toaster oven temperature recommendations by twenty-five degrees to avoid overcooking.

Chapter 3.Tips for Using Your Air fryer

One of the main problems facing families today is the excessive consumption of processed foods and fast foods, which are often high in fat, sugar, and preservatives. One of the best ways to deal with this problem is by learning how to prepare healthy meals at home, but the problem is that cooking at home can be time consuming and requires a lot of equipment. This is where your Breville smart mini-oven comes in. Because it is so easy to use and clean, cooking at home is no longer a problem.

Breville Mini Smart Oven controls are easy to use that even a beginner can become a seasoned home cook in no time. After learning how it works, the whole family will want to join in the fun of cooking quick, easy, and most importantly, healthy meals.

Preparing to Cook

- For the best final result, pat off any excess moisture from the foods. This includes meat that has been soaked in a marinade and foods that have a high level of moisture, such as potatoes.
- You need very little oil when you cook with your air fryer, and some food will not require any oil at all. However, if you are not using any oil, it is a good idea to use a little non-stick cooking spray applied directly to the food or the basket. This will help prevent your creation from sticking to the basket.
- When cutting an ingredient, try to keep the pieces uniform in size; this will ensure even cooking.
- Double check to make sure any fat drippings have been removed from the bottom of the air fryer after the previous use. Allowing fats and oils to accumulate will cause spattering and create smoke.
- When placing foods in the air fryer, remember to place them, so there is plenty of room for air to circulate, even if it means cooking in batches. This will protect the quality of the finished dish and ensure even and proper cooking.
- Preheat the air fryer by setting it to the desired cooking temperature at least three to five minutes before you plan to start cooking.

During Cooking

- Note that recipes and cooking times are an approximation. Your pieces of meat, vegetables, etc. might be a different size, or you may wish to alter the amounts of the ingredients. You might also prefer a different level of doneness. Adjust the cooking times up or down depending on the alterations you make or to suit your individual taste. How closely packed the food is in the air fryer will also impact the amount of time needed for the dish to fully cook.
- Halfway through the cooking time, rotate your food. For smaller items such as fries, this means simply shaking the basket. Larger items should be flipped over.

Always Remember

The air fryer can add an exciting new element to your culinary repertoire. There is no reason you need to stick to traditional "fried" foods. This book will introduce you to additional dishes that can be created in your air fryer. This appliance is meant to be a healthy addition to your kitchen, and with some creativity and experimentation, you can add an incredible variety of fried, roasted, steamed, and baked dishes to your list of culinary creations.

Chapter 4.Breakfast

1.Breakfast Ham Omelet

Preparation Time: 10 minutes
Cooking Time: 10 minutes
Servings: 2
Ingredients:

- 4 large eggs
- 100g ham, cut into small pieces
- ¼ cup milk
- ¾ cup mixed vegetables (white mushrooms, green onions, red pepper)
- ¼ cup mixed cheddar and mozzarella cheese
- 1 tsp. freshly chopped mixed herbs (cilantro and chives)
- Salt and freshly ground pepper to taste

Directions:

1. Combine the eggs and milk in a medium bowl, then add in the remaining ingredients apart from the cheese and mixed herbs and beat well using a fork.
2. Pour the egg mixture into an evenly greased pan, then place it in the basket of your Breville smart air fryer toast oven.
3. Cook for roughly 10 minutes at 350°F or until done to desire.
4. Sprinkle the cheese and mixed herbs on the omelet halfway through cook time.
5. Gently loosen the omelet from the sides of the pan using a spatula.
6. Serve hot!

Nutrition:
Calories: 411 kcal/Cal
Carbs: 14 g
Fat: 39.3 g
Protein: 28 g

2.Crunchy Zucchini Hash Browns

Preparation Time: 30 minutes
Cooking Time: 15 minutes
Servings: 3
Ingredients:

- medium zucchinis, peeled and grated
- 1 tsp. onion powder
- 1 tsp. garlic powder
- tbsp. almond flour
- 1 ½ tsp. chili flakes
- Salt and freshly ground pepper to taste
- 2 tsp. olive oil

Directions:

1.Put the grated zucchini in between layers of kitchen towel and squeeze to drain excess water. Pour 1 teaspoon of oil in a pan, preferably non-stick, over medium heat, and sauté the potatoes for about 3 minutes.
2.Transfer the zucchini to a shallow bowl and let cool. Sprinkle it with the remaining ingredients and mix it until it forms a proper mixture.
3.Transfer the zucchini mixture to a flat plate and pat it down to make 1 compact layer. Put in the fridge and let it sit for 20 minutes.
4.Set your Breville smart air fryer toast oven to 360°F.
5.Meanwhile, take out the flattened zucchini and divide into equal portions using a knife or cookie cutter.
6.Lightly brush your Breville smart air fryer toast oven's basket with the remaining teaspoon of olive oil.
7.Gently place the zucchini pieces into the greased basket and fry for 12-15 minutes, flipping the hash browns halfway through.
8.Enjoy hot!

Nutrition
Calories: 195 kcal/Cal
Carbs: 10.4 g
Fat: 13.1 g
Protein: 9.6 g

3.Breakfast Chicken Strips

Preparation Time: 5 minutes
Cooking Time: 12 minutes
Servings: 4
Ingredients:

- 1 teaspoon paprika
- 1 tablespoon cream
- 1 lb. chicken fillet
- ½ teaspoon salt
- ½ teaspoon black pepper

Directions:
1.Cut the chicken fillet into strips.
2.Sprinkle the chicken fillets with salt and pepper.
3. Preheat the air fryer to 365°Fahrenheit.
4.Place the butter in the air basket tray and add the chicken strips. Cook the chicken strips for 6-minutes.
5.Turn the chicken strips to the other side and cook them for another 5-minutes.
6.After strips are cooked, sprinkle them with cream and paprika, then transfer them to serving plates. Serve warm.
Nutrition:
Calories: 245,
Total Fat: 11.5g,
Carbs: 0.6g,
Protein: 33g

4.Citrus Blueberry Muffins

Preparation Time: 15 minutes
Cooking Time: 15 minutes
Servings: 3-4
Ingredients:
- 2 ½ cups cake flour
- ½ cup sugar
- ¼ cup light cooking oil such as avocado oil
- ½ cup heavy cream
- 1 cup fresh blueberries
- 2 eggs
- Zest and juice from 1 orange
- 1 tsp. pure vanilla extract
- 1 tsp. brown sugar for topping

Directions:
1.Start by combining the oil, heavy cream, eggs, orange juice, and vanilla extract in a large bowl, then set aside.
2.Separately combine the flour and sugar until evenly it's mixed, then pour little by little into the wet ingredients.
3.Combine until well blended but be careful not to over-mix.
4.Preheat your Breville smart air fryer toast oven at 320°F
5.Gently fold the blueberries into the batter and divide into cupcake holders, preferably silicone cupcake holders, as you won't have to grease them. Alternatively, you can use cupcake paper liners on any cupcake holders/ tray you could be having.
6.Sprinkle the tops with the brown sugar and pop the muffins in the fryer.
7.Bake for about 12 minutes. Use a toothpick to check for readiness. When the muffins have evenly browned, and an inserted toothpick comes out clean, they are ready.
8.Take out the muffins and let cool.
9.Enjoy!
Nutrition:
Calories: 289 kcal/Cal,
Carbs: 12.8 g
Fat: 32 g
Protein: 21.1 g

5.PB &J Donuts

Preparation Time: 15 minutes
Cooking Time: 12 minutes
Servings: 4
Ingredients:
For the Donuts:
- 1 ¼ cups all-purpose flour
- ½ tsp. baking soda
- ½ tsp. baking powder
- 1/3 cup sugar
- ½ cup buttermilk
- 1 large egg
- 1 tsp. pure vanilla extract
- 3 tbsp. unsalted, melted and divided into 2+1
- ¾ tsp. salt

For the Glaze:
- 2 tbsp. milk
- ½ cup powdered sugar
- 2 tbsp. smooth peanut butter
- Sea salt to taste

For the Filling:
- ½ cup strawberry or blueberry jelly

Directions:
1.Whisk together all the dry ingredients for the donut in a large bowl.
2.Separately combine the egg, buttermilk, melted butter, and vanilla extract.
3.Create a small well at the center of the dry ingredients and pour in the egg mixture. Use a fork to combine the ingredients, then finish off with a spatula.
4.Place the dough on a floured surface and knead the dough. It will start out sticky, but as you knead, it's going to come together.

5.Roll out the dough to make a ¾ inch thick circle. Use a cookie cutter or the top part of a cup to cut the dough into rounds.
6.Place the donuts on a parchment paper and then into your Breville smart air fryer toast oven. You may have to cook in batches depending on the size of your unit.
7.Cook for 12 minutes at 350°F.
8.Use a pastry bag or squeeze bottle to fill the donuts with jelly.
9.Combine the glaze ingredients and drizzle on top of the donuts.
10.Enjoy!

Nutrition:
Calories: 430 kcal/Cal
Carbs: 66.8 g
Fat: 14.6 g
Protein: 9.1 g

6.Breakfast Baked Apple

Preparation Time: 10 minutes
Cooking Time: 20 minutes
Servings: 2
Ingredients:

- 1 apple
- 2 tbsp. raisins
- 2 tbsp. walnuts, chopped
- ¼ tsp. nutmeg
- ¼ tsp. ground cinnamon
- 1 ½ tsp. margarine
- ¼ cup water

Directions:
1.Start by setting your Breville smart air fryer toast oven to 350°F.
2.Cut the apple in half and gently spoon out some of the flesh.
3.Place the apple halves on your Breville smart air fryer toast ovens frying pan.
4.Mix the raisins, walnuts, nutmeg, cinnamon, and margarine in a bowl and divide equally between the apple halves.
5.Pour the water into the pan and cook for 20 minutes.
6.Enjoy!

Nutrition:
Calories: 161 kcal/Cal
Carbs: 23.7 g
Fat: 7.8 g
Protein: 2.5g

7.Sunny Side up Egg Tarts

Preparation Time: 15 minutes
Cooking Time: 20 minutes
Servings: 2
Ingredients:

- 4 eggs
- ¾ cup shredded Gruyere cheese (or preferred cheese)
- 1 sheet of puff pastry
- Minced chives for topping

Directions:
1.Start by flouring a clean surface, then gently roll out your sheet of puff pastry and divide it into four equal squares.
2.If you have a small Breville smart air fryer toast oven, start with two squares but if it's big enough, go ahead and place the squares on the basket and cook for about 8-10 minutes or until they turn golden brown.
3.Whilst still in the basket, gently make an indentation at the center of each square and sprinkle 2-4 tablespoons of shredded cheese in the well, then crack an egg on top.
4.Cook for 5-10 minutes or to desired doneness.
5.Remove from Breville smart air fryer toast oven, sprinkle with chives, and you are ready to eat!

Nutrition:
Calories: 403 kcal/Cal
Carbs: 10.8 g
Fat: 29.4 g
Protein: 24.6 g

8.Healthy Spinach Scramble

Preparation Time: 8 minutes
Cooking Time: 30 minutes
Servings: 1
Ingredients:

- 3 egg whites
- 1 cup (packed) spinach
- 1 onion, chopped
- 2 tbsp. extra virgin olive oil
- ½ tsp. onion powder
- ½ tsp. garlic powder
- 1 tsp. turmeric powder
- Ground pepper to taste

Directions:
1.Preheat your Breville smart air fryer toast oven to 350°F.

2.Beat the egg whites and oil in a large bowl. Add in the fresh ingredients and mix until well combined, then set the bowl aside.
3.Lightly grease your Breville smart air fryer toast oven's frying pan and transfer the egg mixture into the pan.
4.Cook in the fryer for about 10 minutes or until done to desire.
5.Serve hot.

Nutrition:

Calories: 285 kcal/Cal
Carbs: 12.3 g
Fat: 21.6 g
Protein: 13 g

9.Healthy Vegan Scramble

Preparation Time: 8 minutes
Cooking Time: 30 minutes
Servings: 3
Ingredients:

- 2 large potatoes, cut into cubes
- 1 tofu block, cut into cubes
- 1 broccoli, divided into florets
- 1 large onion, chopped
- 2 tbsp. dark soy sauce
- 2 tbsp. extra virgin olive oil, divided into 1+1
- ½ tsp. onion powder
- ½ tsp. garlic powder
- 1 tsp. turmeric powder
- Ground pepper to taste

Directions:

1.Start by marinating the tofu in 1 tablespoon of olive oil onion, garlic, turmeric, and onion powders, then set aside.
2.Drizzle the potatoes with the remaining tablespoon of olive oil and toss with pepper and cook in the Breville smart air fryer toast oven for 15 minutes at 400°F. Halfway through cook time, toss the potatoes to allow even cooking.
3.Toss the potatoes once more, then mix in the marinated tofu, reserving the leftover liquid, and cook for another 15 minutes at 370°F.
4.Toss the broccoli florets in the leftover marinade. If it's too little, drizzle with some soy sauce and toss to ensure all the florets are evenly covered.
5.When the potato-tofu mixture has 5 minutes of cooking time left, add in the broccoli.
6.Serve hot.

Nutrition:

Calories: 319 kcal/Cal
Carbs: 50.4 g
Fat: 10.9 g,
Protein: 8 g

10.Eggs in Zucchini Nests

Preparation Time: 5 minutes
Cooking Time: 7 minutes
Servings: 4
Ingredients:

- 4 teaspoons butter
- ½ teaspoon paprika
- ½ teaspoon black pepper
- ¼ teaspoon sea salt
- 4-ounces cheddar cheese, shredded
- 4 eggs
- 8-ounces zucchini, grated

Directions:

1.Grate the zucchini and place the butter in ramekins.
2.Add the grated zucchini in ramekins in the shape of nests. Sprinkle the zucchini nests with salt, pepper, and paprika.
3.Beat the eggs and pour over zucchini nests.
4.Top egg mixture with shredded cheddar cheese.
5.Preheat the air fryer basket and cook the dish for 7-minutes.
6.When the zucchini nests are cooked, chill them for 3-minutes and serve them in the ramekins.

Nutrition:

Calories: 221,
Total Fat: 17.7g,
Carbs: 2.9g,
Protein: 13.4g

Chapter 5.Breakfast 2

11.Protein Egg Cups

Preparation Time: 10 minutes
Cooking Time: 9 minutes
Servings: 2
Ingredients:

- 3 eggs, lightly beaten
- 4 tomato slices
- 4 tsp cheddar cheese, shredded
- 2 bacon slices, cooked and crumbled
- Pepper
- Salt

Directions:

1.Spray silicone muffin molds with cooking spray.
2.In a small bowl, whisk the egg with pepper and salt. Preheat the air fryer to 350 F.
3. Pour eggs into the silicone muffin molds. Divide cheese and bacon into molds.
4.Top each with a tomato slice and place in the air fryer basket.
5.Cook for 9 minutes.
6.Serve and enjoy.

Nutrition:
Calories 67
Fat 4 g
Carbohydrates 1 g
Sugar 0.7 g
Protein 5.1 g
Cholesterol 125 mg

12.Pumpkin Pancakes

Preparation Time: 15 minutes
Cooking Time: 12 minutes
Servings: 2
Ingredients:

- 1 square puff pastry
- 3 tablespoons pumpkin filling
- 1 small egg, beaten

Directions:

1.Roll out a square of puff pastry and layer it with pumpkin pie filling, leaving about ¼-inch space around the edges.
2.Cut it up into 8 equal-sized square pieces and coat the edges with a beaten egg.
3.Press "Power Button" of Air Fry Oven and turn the dial to select the "Air Fry" mode.
4.Press the Time button and again turn the dial to set the cooking time to 12 minutes.
5.Don't push the Temp button and rotate the dial to set the temperature at 355 degrees F.
6.Press the "Start/Pause" button to start.
7.When the unit beeps to show that it is preheated, open the lid.
8.Arrange the squares into a greased "Sheet Pan" and insert in the oven.
9.Serve warm.

Nutrition:
Calories 109
Total Fat 6.7 g
Saturated Fat 1.8 g
Cholesterol 34 mg
Sodium 87 mg
Total Carbs 9.8 g
Fiber 0.5 g
Sugar 2.6 g
Protein 2.4 g

13.Shrimp Frittata

Preparation Time: 10 minutes
Cooking Time: 15 minutes
Servings: 2
Ingredients:

- 4 eggs
- ½ teaspoon basil, dried
- Cooking spray
- Salt and black pepper to the taste
- ½ cup rice, cooked
- ½ cup shrimp, cooked, peeled, deveined, and chopped
- ½ cup baby spinach, chopped
- ½ cup Monterey jack cheese, grated

Directions:

1.In a bowl, mix eggs with salt, pepper, and basil and whisk.
2.Grease your air fryer's pan with cooking spray and add rice, shrimp, and spinach.
3.Add egg mix, sprinkle cheese all over and cook in your air fryer at 350 degrees F for 10 minutes.
4.Divide among plates and serve for breakfast.
5.Enjoy!

Nutrition:
Calories 162
Fat 6
Fiber 5
Carbs 8
Protein 4

14.Tuna Sandwiches

Preparation Time: 10 minutes
Cooking Time: 5 minutes
Servings: 2
Ingredients:

- 16 ounces canned tuna, drained
- ¼ cup mayonnaise
- 2 tablespoons mustard
- 1 tablespoon lemon juice
- 2 green onions, chopped
- 3 English muffins, halved
- 3 tablespoons butter
- provolone cheese

Directions:

1.In a bowl, mix tuna with mayo, lemon juice, mustard, and green onions and stir. Grease muffin halves with the butter.
2.Place them in a preheated air fryer and bake them at 350 degrees F for 4 minutes. Spread tuna mix on muffin halves.
3.Top each with provolone cheese, return sandwiches to air fryer, and cook them for 4 minutes.
4.Divide among plates and serve for breakfast right away.
5.Enjoy!

Nutrition:
Calories: 182
Fat: 4
Fiber: 7
Carbs: 8
Protein: 6

15.Cloud Eggs

Preparation Time: 8 minutes
Cooking Time: 4 minutes
Servings: 2
Ingredients:

- 1 teaspoon butter
- 2 eggs

Directions:

1.Separate the eggs and the egg yolks from the egg whites.
2.Then whisk the egg whites with the aid of the hand mixer until the white peaks are strong.
3.After that, spread the butter over the air fryer basket tray.
4.Heat up the air fryer to 300 F.
5.Get the egg white peaks medium clouds in the ready air fryer basket tray.
6.In the Air Fryer, position the basket tray and cook the cloud eggs for two minutes.
7.Take away the basket from the air Fryer after this, place the egg yolks in the middle of each egg cloud, and return the basket to the air fryer.
8.Cook the dish for an extra 2 minutes.
9.Then extract the cooked meal from the basket and serve.

Nutrition:
Calories 80,
Fat 6.3,
Fiber 0,
Carbs 0.3,
Protein 5.6

16.Chicken & Zucchini Omelet

Preparation Time: 15 minutes
Cooking Time: 35 minutes
Servings: 2
Ingredients:

- 4 eggs
- ½ cup milk
- Salt and ground black pepper, as required
- 1 cup cooked chicken, chopped
- 1 cup Cheddar cheese, shredded
- ½ cup fresh chives, chopped
- ¾ cup zucchini, chopped

Directions:

1.In a bowl, add the eggs, milk, salt, and black pepper and beat well.
2.Add the remaining ingredients and stir to combine.
3.Place the mixture into a greased baking pan. Press "Power Button" of Air Fry Oven and turn the dial to select the "Bake" mode.
4.Press the Time button and again turn the dial to set the cooking time to 35 minutes.
5.Now push the Temp button and rotate the dial to set the temperature at 315 degrees F. Press the "Start/Pause" button to start.
6.When the unit beeps to show that it is preheated, open the lid.
7.Arrange pan over the "Wire Rack" and insert in the oven.
8. Cut into equal-sized wedges and serve hot.

Nutrition:
Calories: 209
Total Fat: 13.3 g

Saturated Fat: 6.3 g
Cholesterol: 258 mg
Sodium: 252 mg
Total Carbs: 2.3 g
Fiber: 0.3 g
Sugar: 1.8 g
Protein: 9.8 g

17.Zucchini Fritters

Preparation Time: 15 minutes
Cooking Time: 7 minutes
Servings: 2
Ingredients:

- 10½ oz. zucchini, grated and squeezed
- oz. Halloumi cheese
- ¼ cup all-purpose flour
- 2 eggs
- 1 teaspoon fresh dill, minced
- Salt and ground black pepper, as required

Directions:

1.In a large bowl and mix together all the ingredients. Make a small-sized fritter from the mixture.
2. Press "Power Button" of Air Fry Oven and turn the dial to select the "Air Fry" mode. Press the Time button and again turn the dial to set the cooking time to 7 minutes.
3.Now push the Temp button and rotate the dial to set the temperature at 355 degrees F. Press the "Start/Pause" button to start.
4.When the unit beeps to show that it is preheated, open the lid. Arrange fritters into grease "Sheet Pan" and insert in the oven.
5.Serve warm.

Nutrition:

Calories: 253
Total Fat: 17.2 g
Saturated Fat: 11 g
Cholesterol: 121 mg
Sodium: 333 mg
Total Carbs: 10 g
Fiber: 1.1 g
Sugar: 2.7 g
Protein: 15.2 g

18.Onion Omelet

Preparation Time: 10 minutes
Cooking Time: 15 minutes
Servings: 2
Ingredients:

- 2 eggs
- ¼ teaspoon low-sodium soy sauce
- Ground black pepper, as required
- 1 teaspoon butter
- 1 medium yellow onion, sliced
- ¼ cup Cheddar cheese, grated

Directions:

1.In a skillet, melt the butter over medium heat and cook the onion and cook for about 8-10 minutes.
2. Remove from the heat and set aside to cool slightly.
3. Meanwhile, in a bowl, add the eggs, soy sauce, and black pepper and beat well.
4. Add the cooked onion and gently stir to combine. Place the zucchini mixture into a small baking pan.
5. Press "Power Button" of Air Fry Oven and turn the dial to select the "Air Fry" mode.
6.Press the Time button and again turn the dial to set the cooking time to 5 minutes.
7.Now push the Temp button and rotate the dial to set the temperature at 255 degrees F. Press the "Start/Pause" button to start.
8. When the unit beeps to show that it is preheated.
9. Open the lid. Arrange pan over the "Wire Rack" and insert in the oven.
10. Cut the omelet into 2 portions and serve hot.

Nutrition:

Calories: 222
Total Fat: 15.4 g
Saturated Fat: 6.9 g
Cholesterol: 347 mg
Sodium: 264 mg
Total Carbs: 6.1 g
Fiber: 1.2 g
Sugar: 3.1 g
Protein: 15.3 g

19.Egg Cups with Bacon

Preparation Time: 10 minutes
Cooking Time: 15 minutes
Servings: 4
Ingredients:

- ½ teaspoon paprika
- 1 tablespoon butter
- ¼ teaspoon salt
- ½ teaspoon dried dill

- 2 eggs
- oz. bacon

Directions:

1.In the blender pot, beat the eggs. Paprika, salt, and dried dill are then added. Using the hand blender, carefully mix the egg mixture.
2.Then pour the butter over four ramekins.
3.Cut the bacon and put it in cup shape in ready-made ramekins.
4.Dress the egg mix with bacon in the middle of each ramekin.
5.Put Air fryer at 360 F.
6.Place the ramekins in the Air fryer and cover it.
7.Cook for 15 minutes.
8.When the time is finished, the mixture of eggs and bacon should be delicious.
9.Take out the egg cups and serve.

Nutrition:

Calories 319,
Fat 25.1,
Fiber 0.1,
Carbs 1.2,
Protein 21.4

20.Almond Crust Chicken

Preparation Time: 10 minutes
Cooking Time: 25 minutes
Servings: 2
Ingredients:

- 2 chicken breasts, skinless and boneless
- 1 tbsp Dijon mustard
- 2 tbsp mayonnaise
- ¼ cup almonds
- Pepper
- Salt

Directions:

1.Add almond into the food processor and process until finely ground. Transfer almonds on a plate and set aside.
2.Mix together mustard and mayonnaise and spread over chicken.
3.Coat chicken with almond and place into the air fryer basket and cook at 350 F for 25 minutes
4.Serve and enjoy.

Nutrition:

Calories 409
Fat 22 g
Carbohydrates 6 g
Sugar 1.5 g
Protein 45 g
Cholesterol 134 mg

21.Breakfast Fish Tacos

Preparation Time: 10 minutes
Cooking Time: 13 minutes
Servings: 2
Ingredients:

- big tortillas
- 1 red bell pepper, chopped
- 1 yellow onion, chopped
- 1 cup corn
- white fish fillets, skinless and boneless
- ½ cup salsa
- A handful mixed romaine lettuce, spinach, and radicchio
- 1 tablespoon parmesan, grated

Directions:

1.Put fish fillets in your air fryer and cook at 350 degrees F for 6 minutes.
2.Meanwhile, heat up a pan over medium-high heat, add bell pepper, onion, and corn, stir and cook for 1-2 minutes.
3.Arrange tortillas on a working surface, divide fish fillets, spread salsa over them, divide mixed veggies and mixed greens, and spread parmesan on each at the end.
4. Roll your tacos, place them in a preheated air fryer, and cook at 350 degrees F for 6 minutes more.
5. Divide fish tacos between plates and serve for breakfast.
6.Enjoy!

Nutrition:

Calories: 200
Fat: 3
Fiber: 7
Carbs: 9
Protein: 5

22.Garlic Potatoes with Bacon

Preparation Time: 10 minutes
Cooking Time: 20 minutes
Servings: 2
Ingredients:

- potatoes, peeled and cut into medium cubes
- garlic cloves, minced
- bacon slices, chopped

- 2 rosemary springs, chopped
- 1 tablespoon olive oil
- Salt and black pepper to the taste
- 2 eggs, whisked

Directions:

1.In your air fryer's pan, mix oil with potatoes, garlic, bacon, rosemary, salt, pepper, and eggs, and whisk.

2.Cook potatoes at 400 degrees F for 20 minutes.

3.Divide everything between plates and serve for breakfast.

4. Enjoy!

Nutrition:

Calories: 211
Fat: 3
Fiber: 5
Carbs: 8
Protein: 5

23.Zucchini Squash Mix

Preparation Time: 10 minutes
Cooking Time: 35 minutes
Servings: 2
Ingredients:

- 1 lb zucchini, sliced
- 1 tbsp parsley, chopped
- 1 yellow squash, halved, deseeded, and chopped
- 1 tbsp olive oil
- Pepper
- Salt

Directions:

1.Add all ingredients into the large bowl and mix well.

2.Transfer bowl mixture into the air fryer basket and cook at 400 F for 35 minutes.

3.Serve and enjoy.

Nutrition:

Calories: 49
Fat: 3 g
Carbohydrates: 4 g
Sugar: 2 g
Protein: 1.5 g
Cholesterol: 0 mg

Chapter 6.Breakfast 3

24.Special Corn Flakes Casserole

Preparation Time: 10 minutes
Cooking Time: 18 Minutes
Servings: 5
Ingredients:

- 1/3 cup milk
- 1 tbsp. cream cheese; whipped
- 1/4 tsp. nutmeg; ground
- 1/4 cup blueberries
- 1 ½ cups corn flakes; crumbled
- 3 tsp. sugar
- 2 eggs; whisked
- bread slices

Directions:
1.In a bowl, mix eggs with sugar, nutmeg, and milk and whisk well.
2.In another bowl, mix cream cheese with blueberries and whisk well.
3.Put corn flakes in a third bowl.
4.Spread blueberry mix on each bread slice; then dip in eggs mix and dredge in corn flakes at the end.
5.Place bread in your air fryer's basket; heat up at 400 °F and bake for 8 minutes.
6.Divide among plates and serve for breakfast.
Nutrition:
Calories: 300;
Fat: 5;
Fiber: 7;
Carbs: 16;
Protein: 4

25.Protein Rich Egg White Omelet

Preparation Time: 10 minutes
Cooking Time: 25 Minutes
Servings: 4
Ingredients:

- 1 cup egg whites
- 1/4 cup mushrooms; chopped
- 2 tbsp. chives; chopped
- 1/4 cup tomato; chopped
- 2 tbsp. skim milk
- Salt and black pepper to the taste

Directions:
1.In a bowl, mix egg whites with tomato, milk, mushrooms, chives, salt, and pepper.
2.Whisk well and pour into your air fryer's pan. Cook at 320 °F for 15 minutes.
3.Cool omelet down, slice, divide among plates, and serve.
Nutrition:
Calories: 100;
Fat: 3;
Fiber: 6;
Carbs: 7;
Carbs: 4

26.Shrimp Sandwiches

Preparation Time: 10 minutes
Cooking Time: 15 Minutes
Servings: 4
Ingredients:

- 1 ¼ cups cheddar; shredded
- 2 tbsp. green onions; chopped.
- whole wheat bread slices
- oz. canned tiny shrimp; drained
- 1 tbsp. mayonnaise
- 2 tbsp. butter; soft

Directions:
1.In a bowl, mix shrimp with cheese, green onion, and mayo and stir well.
2.Spread this on half of the bread slices; top with the other bread slices, cut into halves diagonally, and spread butter on top.
3.Place sandwiches in your air fryer and cook at 350 °F for 5 minutes. Divide shrimp sandwiches between plates and serve them for breakfast.
Nutrition:
Calories: 162;
Fat: 3;
Fiber: 7;
Carbs: 12; Protein: 4

27.Breakfast Soufflé

Preparation Time: 10 minutes
Cooking Time: 18 Minutes
Servings: 4
Ingredients:

- 4 eggs; whisked
- 1 tbsp. heavy cream
- 2 tbsp. parsley; chopped.
- 2 tbsp. chives; chopped.
- A pinch of red chili pepper; crushed
- Salt and black pepper to the taste

Directions:

1.In a bowl, mix eggs with salt, pepper, heavy cream, red chili pepper, parsley, and chives; stir well and divide into 4 soufflé dishes.
2.Arrange dishes in your air fryer and cook soufflés at 350 °F for 8 minutes. Serve them hot.

Nutrition: Calories:
300; Fat: 7;
Fiber: 9;
Carbs: 15;
Protein: 6

28.Fried Tomato Quiche

Preparation Time: 10 minutes
Cooking Time: 40 Minutes
Servings: 1
Ingredients:

- 1 tbsp. yellow onion; chopped.
- 1/2 cup gouda cheese; shredded
- 1/4 cup tomatoes; chopped.
- 2 eggs
- 1/4 cup milk
- Salt and black pepper to the taste
- Cooking spray

Directions:
1.Grease a ramekin with cooking spray.
2.Crack eggs, add onion, milk, cheese, tomatoes, salt, and pepper, and stir. Add this to your air fryer's pan and cook at 340 °F for 30 minutes.

Nutrition:
Calories: 241;
Fat: 6;
Fiber: 8;
Carbs: 14;
Protein: 6

29.Breakfast Spanish Omelet

Preparation Time: 10 minutes
Cooking Time: 20 Minutes
Servings: 4
Ingredients:

- eggs
- 1/2 chorizo; chopped
- 1 tbsp. parsley; chopped.
- 1 tbsp. feta cheese; crumbled
- 1 potato; peeled and cubed
- 1/2 cup corn
- 1 tbsp. olive oil
- Salt and black pepper to the taste

Directions:
1.Heat up your air fryer at 350 °F and add oil.
2.Add chorizo and potatoes; stir and brown them for a few seconds.
3.In a bowl, mix eggs with corn, parsley, cheese, salt and pepper, and whisk.
4.Pour this over chorizo and potatoes; spread and cook for 5 minutes. Divide omelet between plates and serve for breakfast.

Nutrition:
Calories: 300;
Fat: 6;
Fiber: 9;
Carbs: 12;
Protein: 6

30.Scrambled Pancake Hash

Preparation Time: 5 minutes
Cooking Time: 9 minutes
Servings: 7
Ingredients:

- 1 egg
- ¼ cup heavy cream
- 2 tablespoons butter
- 1 cup coconut flour
- 1 teaspoon ground ginger
- 1 teaspoon salt
- 1 tablespoon apple cider vinegar
- 1 teaspoon baking soda

Directions:
1. Combine the salt, baking soda, ground ginger, and flour in a mixing bowl. In a separate bowl crack, the egg into it.
2. Add butter and heavy cream.
3. Mix well using a hand mixer. Combine the liquid and dry mixtures and stir until smooth.
4. Preheat your air fryer to 400°Fahrenheit. Pour the pancake mixture into the air fryer basket tray.
5. Cook the pancake hash for 4-minutes.
6. After this, scramble the pancake hash well and continue to cook for another 5-minutes more.
7. When the dish is cooked, transfer it to serving plates, and serve hot!

Nutrition:
Calories: 178,
Total Fat: 13.3g,
Carbs: 10.7g,
Protein: 4.4g

31.Onion Frittata

Preparation Time: 20 minutes
Cooking Time: 30 Minutes
Servings: 6
Ingredients:

- 4 eggs; whisked
- 1 tbsp. olive oil
- 1 lb. small potatoes; chopped
- 1 oz. cheddar cheese; grated
- 1/2 cup sour cream
- yellow onions; chopped
- Salt and black pepper to the taste

Directions:

1.In a large bowl, mix eggs with potatoes, onions, salt, pepper, cheese, and sour cream and whisk well.
2.Grease your air fryer's pan with the oil, add eggs mix; place in the air fryer and cook for 20 minutes at 320 degrees F. Slice frittata, divide among plates and serve for breakfast.

Nutrition:

Calories: 231;
Fat: 5;
Fiber: 7;
Carbs: 8;
Protein: 4

32.Pea Tortilla

Preparation Time: 10 minutes
Cooking Time: 17 Minutes
Servings: 8
Ingredients:

- 1/2 lb. baby peas
- 1 ½ cup yogurt
- 4 eggs
- 1/2 cup mint; chopped.
- tbsp. butter
- Salt and black pepper to the taste

Directions:

1.Heat up a pan that fits your air fryer with the butter over medium heat, add peas, stir and cook for a couple of minutes.
2.Meanwhile, in a bowl, mix half of the yogurt with salt, pepper, eggs, and mint and whisk well.
3.Pour this over the peas, toss, introduce in your air fryer and cook at 350 °F for 7 minutes. Spread the rest of the yogurt over your tortilla; slice and serve.

Nutrition:

Calories: 192;
Fat: 5;
Fiber: 4;
Carbs: 8;
Protein: 7

33.Mushroom Quiches

Preparation Time: 10 minutes
Cooking Time: 20 Minutes
Servings: 4
Ingredients:

- button mushrooms; chopped.
- 1 tbsp. ham; chopped
- 4 eggs
- 1 tbsp. flour
- 1 tbsp. butter; soft
- 9-inch pie dough
- 1/2 tsp. thyme; dried
- 1/4 cup Swiss cheese; grated
- 1 small yellow onion; chopped.
- 1/3 cup heavy cream
- A pinch of nutmeg; ground
- Salt and black pepper to the taste

Directions:

1.Dust a working surface with the flour and roll the pie dough.
2.Press in on the bottom of the pie pan your air fryer has.
3.In a bowl, mix butter with mushrooms, ham, onion, eggs, heavy cream, salt, pepper, thyme, and nutmeg and whisk well.
4.Add this over pie crust, spread, sprinkle Swiss cheese all over and place the pie pan in your air fryer.
5.Cook your quiche at 400 °F for 10 minutes. Slice and serve for breakfast.

Nutrition:

Calories: 212;
Fat: 4;
Fiber: 6;
Carbs: 7;
Protein: 7

34.Walnuts Pear Oatmeal

Preparation Time: 10 minutes
Cooking Time: 17 Minutes
Servings: 4
Ingredients:

- 1 tbsp. butter; soft
- 1/4 cups brown sugar
- 1 cup water
- 1/2 cup raisins

- 1/2 tsp. cinnamon powder
- 1 cup rolled oats
- 1/2 cup walnuts; chopped.
- 2 cups pear; peeled and chopped.

Directions:

1.In a heatproof dish that fits your air fryer; mix milk with sugar, butter, oats, cinnamon, raisins, pears, and walnuts; stir,

2.introduce in your fryer and cook at 360 °F for 12 minutes.

3.Divide into bowls and serve.

Nutrition:

Calories: 230;
Fat: 6;
Fiber: 11;
Carbs: 20;
Protein: 5

35.Breakfast Raspberry Rolls

Preparation Time: 10 minutes
Cooking Time: 50 Minutes
Servings: 6
Ingredients:

- 1 cup milk
- 1/4 cup sugar
- 1 egg
- tbsp. butter
- ¼ cups flour
- tsp. yeast

For the filling:

- oz. cream cheese; soft
- oz. raspberries
- 1 tsp. vanilla extract
- tbsp. sugar
- 1 tbsp. cornstarch
- Zest from 1 lemon; grated

Directions:

1.In a bowl; mix flour with sugar and yeast and stir.

2.Add milk and egg, stir until you obtain a dough, leave it aside to rise for 30 minutes, transfer the dough to a working surface and roll well.

3.In a bowl, mix cream cheese with sugar, vanilla, and lemon zest; stir well and spread over dough.

4.In another bowl, mix raspberries with cornstarch, stir and spread over cream cheese mixture.

5.Roll your dough, cut into medium pieces, place them in your air fryer; spray them with cooking spray, and cook them at 350 °F for 30 minutes. Serve your rolls for breakfast.

Nutrition:

Calories: 261;
Fat: 5;
Fiber: 8;
Carbs: 9;
Protein: 6

36.Bread Pudding

Preparation Time: 10 minutes
Cooking Time: 32 Minutes
Servings: 4
Ingredients:

- 1/2 lb. white bread; cubed
- 3/4 cup milk
- 3/4 cup water
- 1 tsp. cinnamon powder
- 1 ⅓ cup flour
- 3/5 cup brown sugar
- 1 tsp. cornstarch
- 1/2 cup apple; peeled; cored, and roughly chopped.
- 1 tbsp. honey
- 1 tsp. vanilla extract
- oz. soft butter

Directions:

1.In a bowl, mix bread with apple, milk with water, honey, cinnamon, vanilla, and cornstarch and whisk well.

2.In a separate bowl, mix flour with sugar and butter and stir until you obtain a crumbled mixture.

3.Press half of the crumble mix on the bottom of your air fryer; add bread and apple mix, add the rest of the crumble and cook everything at 350 °F for 22 minutes. Divide bread pudding between plates and serve.

Nutrition:

Calories: 261;
Fat: 7; Fiber: 7;
Carbs: 8;
Protein: 5

37.Cream Cheese Oats

Preparation Time: 10 minutes
Cooking Time: 35 Minutes
Servings: 4
Ingredients:

- 1 cup steel oats
- 2 cups milk

- 1 tbsp. butter
- tbsp. white sugar
- oz. cream cheese; soft
- 3/4 cup raisins
- 1 tsp. cinnamon powder
- 1/4 cup brown sugar

Directions:

1.Heat up a pan that fits your air fryer with the butter over medium heat, add oats, stir and toast them for 3 minutes.
2.Add milk and raisins; stir, introduce in your air fryer and cook at 350 °F for 20 minutes.
3.Meanwhile, in a bowl, mix cinnamon with brown sugar and stir.
4.In a second bowl, mix white sugar with cream cheese and whisk. Divide oats into bowls and top each with cinnamon and cream cheese.

Nutrition:

Calories: 152;
Fat: 6;
Fiber: 6;
Carbs: 25;
Protein: 7

38.Bread Rolls

Preparation Time: 10 minutes
Cooking Time: 22 Minutes
Servings: 4
Ingredients:

- 3 potatoes; boiled; peeled and mashed
- 1/2 tsp. turmeric powder
- curry leaf springs
- 1/2 tsp. mustard seeds
- bread slices; white parts only
- 1 coriander bunch; chopped.
- green chilies; chopped
- small yellow onions; chopped.
- 2 tbsp. olive oil
- Salt and black pepper to the taste

Directions:

1.Heat up a pan with 1 tsp. oil; add mustard seeds, onions, curry leaves, and turmeric, stir and cook for a few seconds.
2.Add mashed potatoes, salt, pepper, coriander, and chilies, stir well; take off the heat and cool it down.
3.Divide potatoes mix into 8 parts and shape ovals using your wet hands.
4.Wet bread slices with water; press in order to drain excess water and keep one slice in your palm.
5.Add a potato oval over bread slice and wrap it around it.
6.Repeat with the rest of the potato mix and bread.
7.Heat up your air fryer at 400 degrees F; add the rest of the oil, add bread rolls; cook them for 12 minutes. Divide bread rolls between plates and serve for breakfast.

Nutrition:

Calories: 261;
Fat: 6;
Fiber: 9;
Carbs: 12;
Protein: 7

Chapter 7.Lunch

39.Sweet & Sour Chicken Skewer

Preparation Time: 10 minutes
Cooking Time: 18 minutes
Servings: 4
Ingredients:

- 1 lb. of chicken tenders
- ¼ teaspoon of pepper
- garlic cloves, minced
- 1 ½ tablespoons soy sauce
- 2 tablespoons pineapple juice
- 1 tablespoon sesame oil
- ½ teaspoon ginger, minced

Directions:
1.Preheat your air fryer to 390˚Fahrenheit.
2.Combine ingredients in a bowl, except for the chicken.
3.Skewer the chicken tenders, then place in a bowl and marinate for 2-hours.
4.Add tenders to the air fryer and cook for 18-minutes.
5.Serve hot!
Nutrition
Calories: 673,
Total Fat: 29g,
Carbs: 9g,
Protein: 39g

40.Sweet Potato Chips

Preparation Time: 5 minutes
Cooking Time: 10 minutes.
Servings: 4
Ingredients:

- large sweet potatoes, cut into strips 25 mm thick
- 15 ml of oil
- 10g of salt
- 2g black pepper
- 2g of paprika
- 2g garlic powder
- 2g onion powder

Directions:
1.Cut the sweet potatoes into strips 25 mm thick.
2.Preheat the air fryer for a few minutes.
3.Add the cut sweet potatoes in a large bowl and mix with the oil until the potatoes are all evenly coated.
4.Sprinkle salt, black pepper, paprika, garlic powder, and onion powder. Mix well.
5.Place the French fries in the preheated baskets and cook for 10 minutes at 205°C. Be sure to shake the baskets halfway through cooking.
Nutrition: Calories: 130
Fat: 0g
Carbohydrates: 29g
Protein: 2g
Sugar: 9g
Cholesterol: 0mg

41.Cajun Style French Fries

Preparation Time: 30 minutes
Cooking Time: 28 minutes.
Servings: 4
Ingredients:

- reddish potatoes, peeled and cut into strips of 76 x 25 mm
- 1 liter of cold water
- 15 ml of oil
- 7g of Cajun seasoning
- 1g cayenne pepper
- Tomato sauce or ranch sauce to serve

Directions:
1.Cut the potatoes into 76 x 25 mm strips and soak them in water for 15 minutes.
2.Drain the potatoes, rinse with cold, dry water with paper towels.
3.Preheat the air fryer, set it to 195°C.
4.Add oil and spices to the potatoes until they are completely covered.
5.Add the potatoes to the preheated air fryer and set the timer to 28 minutes.
6.Be sure to shake the baskets in the middle of cooking
7.Remove the baskets from the air fryer when you have finished cooking and season the fries with salt and pepper.
8.Serve with tomato sauce or ranch sauce.
Nutrition:
Calories: 156
Fat: 8.01g
Carbohydrate: 20.33g
Protein: 1.98g
Sugar: 0.33g
Cholesterol: 0mg

42.Fried Zucchini

Preparation Time: 10 minutes.
Cooking Time: 8 minutes.
Servings: 4
Ingredients:

- medium zucchinis, cut into strips 19 mm thick
- 60g all-purpose flour
- 12g of salt
- 2g black pepper
- beaten eggs
- 15 ml of milk
- 84g Italian seasoned breadcrumbs
- 25g grated Parmesan cheese
- Nonstick Spray Oil
- Ranch sauce to serve

Directions:
1.Cut the zucchini into strips 19 mm thick.
2.Mix with the flour, salt, and pepper on a plate. Mix the eggs and milk in a separate dish. Put breadcrumbs and Parmesan cheese in another dish.
3.Cover each piece of zucchini with flour, then dip them in egg and pass them through the crumbs. Leave aside.
4.Preheat the air fryer, set it to 175°C.
5.Place the covered zucchini in the preheated air fryer and spray with oil spray. Set the timer to 8 minutes and press Start
6.Pause.
7.Be sure to shake the baskets in the middle of cooking.
8.Serve with tomato sauce or ranch sauce.
Nutrition:
Calories: 67
Fat: 4.1g
Carbohydrates: 4.5g
Protein: 3.3g
Sugar: 1.47g
Cholesterol: 20.7mg

43.Fried Avocado

Preparation Time: 15 minutes.
Cooking Time: 10 minutes.
Servings: 2
Ingredients:

- avocados cut into wedges 25 mm thick
- 50g Pan crumbs bread
- 2g garlic powder
- 2g onion powder
- 1g smoked paprika
- 1g cayenne pepper
- Salt and pepper to taste
- 60g all-purpose flour
- eggs, beaten
- Nonstick Spray Oil
- Tomato sauce or ranch sauce to serve

Directions:
1.Cut the avocados into 25 mm thick pieces.
2.Combine the crumbs, garlic powder, onion powder, smoked paprika, cayenne pepper, and salt in a bowl.
3.Separate each wedge of avocado in the flour, then dip the beaten eggs and stir in the breadcrumb mixture.
4.Preheat the air fryer.
5.Place the avocados in the preheated air fryer baskets, spray with oil spray, and cook at 205°C for 10 minutes. Turn the fried avocado halfway through cooking and sprinkle with cooking oil.
6.Serve with tomato sauce or ranch sauce.
Nutrition:
Calories: 96
Fat: 8.8g
Carbohydrates: 5.12g
Protein: 1.2g
Sugar: 0.4g
Cholesterol: 0mg

44.Vegetables In air Fryer

Preparation Time: 20 minutes.
Cooking Time: 30 minutes.
Servings: 2
Ingredients:

- potatoes
- 1 zucchini
- 1 onion
- 1 red pepper
- 1 green pepper

Directions:
1.Cut the potatoes into slices.
2.Cut the onion into rings.
3.Cut the zucchini slices
4.Cut the peppers into strips.
5.Put all the ingredients in the bowl and add a little salt, ground pepper, and some extra virgin olive oil.
6.Mix well.

7.Pass to the basket of the air fryer.
8.Select 1600C, 30 minutes.
9.Check that the vegetables are to your liking.
Nutrition:
Calories: 135
Fat: 11g
Carbohydrates: 8g
Protein: 1g
Sugar: 2g
Cholesterol: 0mg

45.Mushrooms Stuffed with Tomato

Preparation Time: 5 minutes.
Cooking Time: 50 minutes.
Servings: 4
Ingredients:

- large mushrooms
- 250g of minced meat
- cloves of garlic
- Extra virgin olive oil
- Salt
- Ground pepper
- Flour, beaten egg, and breadcrumbs
- Frying oil
- Fried Tomato Sauce

Directions:
1.Remove the stem from the mushrooms and chop it. Peel the garlic and chop. Put some extra virgin olive oil in a pan and add the garlic and mushroom stems.
2.Sauté and add the minced meat. Sauté well until the meat is well cooked and season.
3.Fill the mushrooms with the minced meat.
4.Press well and take the freezer for 30 minutes.
5.Pass the mushrooms with flour, beaten egg, and breadcrumbs. Beaten egg and breadcrumbs.
6.Place the mushrooms in the basket of the air fryer.
7.Select 20 minutes, 1800C.
8.Distribute the mushrooms once cooked in the dishes.
9.Heat the tomato sauce and cover the stuffed mushrooms.
Nutrition:
Calories: 160
Fat: 7.96g
Carbohydrates: 19.41g
Protein: 7.94g
Sugar: 9.19g
Cholesterol: 0mg

46.Spiced Potato Wedges

Preparation Time: 15 minutes
Cooking Time: 40 minutes.
Servings: 4
Ingredients:

- medium potatoes
- Salt
- Ground pepper
- Garlic powder
- Aromatic herbs, the one we like the most
- 1 tbsp extra virgin olive oil
- 1 tbsp breadcrumbs or chickpea flour

Directions:
1.Put the unpeeled potatoes in a pot with boiling water and a little salt.
2.Let cook for 5 minutes. Drain and let cool. Cut into thick segments without peeling.
3.Put the potatoes in a bowl and add salt, pepper, garlic powder, the aromatic herb that we have chosen oil, and breadcrumbs or chickpea flour.
4.Stir well and leave for 15 minutes. Pass to the basket of the air fryer and select 20 minutes, 1800C.
5.From time to time shake the basket so that the potatoes mix and change position. Check that they are tender.
Nutrition:
Calories: 121
Fat: 3g
Carbohydrates: 19g
Protein: 2g
Sugar: 0g
Cholesterol: 0mg

47.Egg Stuffed Zucchini Balls

Preparation Time: 15 minutes.
Cooking Time: 45-60 minutes.
Servings: 4
Ingredients:

- zucchinis
- 1 onion
- 1 egg
- 120g of grated cheese
- 4 eggs
- Salt
- Ground pepper

- Flour

Directions:

1.Chop the zucchini and onion in the air fryer, 10 seconds speed 8, in the Cuisine with the kneader chopper at speed 10 about 15 seconds, or we can chop the onion by hand and the zucchini grate. No matter how you do it, the important thing is that the zucchini and onion are as small as possible.
2.Put in a bowl and add the cheese and the egg. Pepper and bind well.
3.Incorporate the flour until you have a very brown dough with which you can wrap the eggs without problems.
4.Cook the eggs and peel.
5.Cover the eggs with the zucchini dough and pass through the flour.
6.Place the four balls in the basket of the air fryer and paint with oil.
7.Select 1800C and leave for 45 to 60 minutes or until you see that the balls are crispy on the outside.
8.Serve over a layer of mayonnaise or aioli.

Nutrition:

Calories: 23
Fat: 0.5g
Carbohydrates: 2g
Protein: 1.8g
Sugar: 0g
Cholesterol: 15mg

48.Vegetables with Provolone

Preparation Time: 10 minutes.
Cooking Time: 30 minutes.
Servings: 4
Ingredients:

- 1 bag of 400g of frozen tempura vegetables
- Extra virgin olive oil
- Salt
- 1 slice of provolone cheese

Directions:

1.Put the vegetables in the basket of the air fryer. Add some strands of extra virgin olive oil and close.
2.Select 20 minutes, 2000C.
3.Pass the vegetables to a clay pot and place the provolone cheese on top.
4.Take to the oven, 1800C, about 10 minutes or so or until you see that the cheese has melted to your liking.

Nutrition:

Calories: 104
Fat: 8g
Carbohydrates: 0g
Protein: 8g
Sugar: 0g
Cholesterol: 0mg

49.Spicy Potatoes

Preparation Time: 10 minutes.
Cooking Time: 30 minutes.
Servings: 4
Ingredients:

- 400g potatoes
- 1 tbsp spicy paprika
- 1 tbsp olive oil
- Caspary or cottage cheese
- Salt to taste

Directions:

1.Wash the potatoes with a brush. Unpeeled, cut vertically in a crescent shape, about 1 finger thick. Place the potatoes in a bowl and cover with water. Let stand for about half an hour.
2.Preheat the air fryer. Set the timer to 5 minutes and the temperature to 2000C.
3.Drain the water from the potatoes and dry with paper towels or a clean cloth. Put them back in the bowl and pour the oil, salt, and paprika over them. Mix well with your hands so that all of them are covered evenly with the spice mixture. Pour the spiced potatoes into the basket of the air fryer. Set the timer for 30 minutes and press the power button. Stir the potatoes in half the time.
4.Remove the potatoes from the air fryer, place on a plate.
5.Serve with cheese and sauce.

Nutrition:

Calories: 153
Fat: 4g
Carbohydrates: 26
Protein: 3g
Sugar: 0g
Cholesterol: 5mg

50.Butter Glazed Carrots

Preparation Time: 20 Minutes
Cooking Time: 15 minutes
Servings: 4
Ingredients:

- Baby carrots-2 cups
- Brown sugar-1 tbsps
- Butter; melted-1/2 tbsps
- Salt and black pepper- a pinch

Directions:

1.Take a baking dish suitable to fit in your air fryer.
2.Toss carrots with sugar, butter, salt, and black peppers in that baking dish.
3.Place this dish in the air fryer basket and seal the fryer.
4.Cook the carrots for 10 minutes at 3500 F on Air fryer mode.
5.Enjoy.

Nutrition:

calories 151,
fat 2,
fiber 4,
carbs 14,
protein 4

51.Roasted Cauliflower with Nuts & Raisins

Preparation Time: 5 minutes
Cooking Time: 15 minutes
Servings: 4
Ingredients:

- 1 small cauliflower head, cut into florets
- 2 tablespoons pine nuts, toasted
- 2 tablespoons raisins, soak in boiling water and drain
- 1 teaspoon curry powder
- ½ teaspoon sea salt
- 1 tablespoons olive oil

Directions:

1.Preheat your air fryer to 320°Fahrenheit for 2-minutes.
2.Add ingredients into a bowl and toss to combine.
3.Add the cauliflower mixture to the air fryer basket and cook for 15-minutes.

Nutrition

Calories: 264,
Total Fat: 26g,
Carbs: 8g,
Protein: 2g

Chapter 8.Lunch 2

52.Korean Barbeque Beef

Preparation Time: 15 minutes
Cooking Time: 30 minutes
Servings: 4
Ingredients:

- 1 Lb. flank steak
- 1/4 Cup corn starch
- 1 Tablespoon Pompeian oil
- 1/2 Cup soy sauce
- 1/2 Cup brown sugar
- 1 Tablespoons Pompeian while vinegar
- 1 Tablespoon garlic (crushed)
- ½ Tablespoon sesame seeds
- 1 Tablespoon corn starch
- 1 Tablespoon water

Directions:

1.The steak should be sliced into thin pieces and rubbed with corn starch and oil.
2.The air fryer toaster oven should be preheated at 390°F for 5 min. The basket should be covered by aluminum foil.
3.The steaks are placed in the basket and heated for 20 min with intermittent flipping.
4.In the meantime, all other ingredients are heated in a pan except water and cornstarch in medium heat to form the sauce.
5.The sauce should be heated until reduced to half.
6.The sauce should be poured over the steak and served with green beans and cooked rice.

Nutrition

Calories: 487 kcal/Cal
Fat: 10 g
Carbs: 32 g
Protein: 39g

53.Beef Burgers

Preparation Time: 5 minutes
Cooking Time: 15 minutes
Servings: 4
Ingredients

- Ground beef patties
- ¼ Tablespoon black pepper
- Slices sharp cheddar cheese
- 1/2 Cup onion (sliced)
- 1/2 Cup tomato (sliced)
- 1 Tablespoon pickles
- Leaves lettuce
- ½ Tablespoon mustard
- hamburger Buns

Directions

1.The beef patties are rubbed with black pepper.
2.The air fryer toaster oven should be preheated at 375F for 5 min. The basket should be covered by aluminum foil.
3. The patties are placed in the basket and heated for 10 min with intermittent flipping.
4.One slice of cheese is placed on each patty and heated for another 2 min.
5. One cooked patty is placed on one bun to which are added lettuce leaves, pickles, onion, and mustard and covered by another bun.
6.Thus, the burger gets ready to be served.

Nutrition

Calories: 240 kcal/Cal
Fat: 6g
Carbs: 11 g
Protein: 16g

54.Chicken Pot Pie

Preparation Time: 10 minutes
Cooking Time: 17 minutes
Servings: 6
Ingredients

- 1 tbsp. olive oil
- 1-pound chicken breast cubed
- 1 tbsp. garlic powder
- 1 tbsp. thyme
- 1 tbsp. pepper
- 1 cup chicken broth
- oz. bag frozen mixed vegetables
- large potatoes cubed
- oz. Can cream of chicken soup
- 1 cup heavy cream
- 1 pie crust
- 1 egg 1 tbsp. water

Directions

1.Hit Sauté on the Breville smart Crispy and add chicken and olive oil.
2.Sauté chicken for 5 minutes, then stir in spices.
3.Pour in the broth along with vegetables and cream of chicken soup
4.Put on the pressure-cooking lid and seal it.

5.Hit the "Pressure Button" and select 10 minutes of cooking time, then press "Start."
6.Once the Breville smart beeps, do a quick release and remove its lid.
7.Remove the lid and stir in cream.
8.Hit sauté and cook for 2 minutes.
9.Enjoy!

Nutrition

Calories: 568 kcal/Cal
Fat: 31.1g
Carbohydrates: 50.8g
Fiber: 3.9g
Protein: 23.4g

55.Chicken Casserole

Preparation Time: 10 Minutes
Cooking Time: 9 minutes
Servings: 6

Ingredients

- cup chicken, shredded
- oz. bag egg noodles
- 1/2 large onion
- 1/2 cup chopped carrots
- 1/4 cup frozen peas
- 1/4 cup frozen broccoli pieces
- stalks celery chopped
- cup chicken broth
- 1 teaspoon garlic powder
- Salt and pepper to taste
- 1 cup cheddar cheese, shredded
- 1 package French's onions
- 1/4 c sour cream
- 1 can cream of chicken and mushroom soup

Directions

1.Add chicken, broth, black pepper, salt, garlic powder, vegetables, and egg noodles to the Breville smart.
2.Put on the pressure-cooking lid and seal it.
3.Hit the "Pressure Button" and select 4 minutes of cooking time, then press "Start."
4.Once the Breville smart beeps, do a quick release and remove its lid.
5.Stir in cheese, 1/3 of French's onions, can of soup, and sour cream.
6.Mix well and spread the remaining onion on top.
7.Put on the Air Fryer lid and seal it.
8.Hit the "Air fryer Button" and select 5 minutes of cooking time, then press "Start."
9.Once the Breville smart beeps, remove its lid.
10. Serve.

Nutrition

Calories: 494 kcal/Cal
Fat: 19.1g
Carbohydrates: 29g
Fiber: 2.6g
Protein: 48.9g

56.Ranch Chicken Wings

Preparation Time: 10 minutes
Cooking Time: 35 minutes
Servings: 6

Ingredients

- chicken wings
- 1 tablespoon olive oil
- 1 cup chicken broth
- 1/4 cup butter
- 1/2 cup Red Hot Sauce
- 1/4 teaspoon Worcestershire sauce
- 1 tablespoon white vinegar
- 1/4 teaspoon cayenne pepper
- 1/8 teaspoon garlic powder
- Seasoned salt to taste
- Ranch dressing for dipping Celery for garnish

Directions

1.Set the Air Fryer Basket in the Breville smart and pour the broth in it.
2.Spread the chicken wings in the basket and put on the pressure-cooking lid.
3.Hit the "Pressure Button" and select 10 minutes of cooking time, then press "Start."
4.Meanwhile, prepare the sauce and add butter, vinegar, cayenne pepper, garlic powder, Worcestershire sauce, and hot sauce in a small saucepan.
5.Cook this sauce for 5 minutes on medium heat until it thickens.
6.Once the Breville smart beeps, do a quick release and remove its lid.
7.Remove the wings and empty the Breville smart.
8.Toss the wings with oil, salt, and black pepper.
9.Set the Air Fryer Basket in the Breville smart and arrange the wings in it.
10. Put on the Air Fryer lid and seal it.
11. Hit the "Air Fryer Button" and select 20 minutes of cooking time, then press "Start."

12. Once the Breville smart air fryer beeps, remove its lid.
13. Transfer the wings to the sauce and mix well.
14. Serve.

Nutrition

Calories: 414
Fat: 31.6g
Carbohydrates 11.2g
Fiber: 0.3g
Protein: 20.4g

57.Tofu Sushi Burrito

Preparation Time: 5 minutes
Cooking Time: 15 minutes
Servings: 2

Ingredients

- ¼ block extra firm tofu, pressed and sliced
- 1 tbsp. low-sodium soy sauce
- ¼ tsp. ground ginger
- ¼ tsp. garlic powder
- Sriracha sauce, to taste
- 2 cups cooked sushi rice
- sheets nori

Filling:

- ¼ avocado, sliced
- 1 tbsp mango, sliced
- 1 green onion, finely chopped
- 1 tbsp. pickled ginger
- 2 tbsp. panko breadcrumbs

Directions

1.Whisk ginger, garlic, soy sauce, sriracha sauce, and tofu in a large bowl.
2.Let them marinate for 10 minutes, then transfer them to the air fryer basket.
3.Return the fryer basket to the air fryer and cook on air fry mode for 15 minutes at 370°F.
4.Toss the tofu cubes after 8 minutes, then resume cooking.
5.Spread a nori sheet on a work surface and top it with a layer of sushi rice.
6.Place tofu and half of the other filling ingredients over the rice.
7.Roll the sheet tightly to secure the filling inside.
8.Repeat the same steps to make another sushi roll.
9.Enjoy!

Nutrition

Calories: 372 kcal/Cal
Fat: 11.8 g
Carbohydrates: 45.8 g
Fiber: 0.6 g
Protein: 34 g

58.Rosemary Brussels Sprouts

Preparation Time: 5 minutes
Cooking Time: 13 minutes
Servings: 2

Ingredients

- 1 tbsp. olive oil
- garlic cloves, minced
- ½ tsp. salt
- ¼ tsp. pepper
- 1 lb. Brussels sprouts, trimmed and halved
- ½ cup panko breadcrumbs
- 1 ½ tsp. fresh rosemary, minced

Directions

1.Let your air fryer preheat at 350°F.
2.Mix oil, garlic, salt, and pepper in a bowl and heat for 30 seconds in the microwave.
3.Add 2 tablespoons of this mixture to the Brussels sprouts in a bowl and mix well to coat.
4.Spread the sprouts in the air fryer basket.
5.Return the fryer basket to the air fryer and cook on air fry mode for 5 minutes at 220°F.
6.Toss the sprouts well and continue air frying for 8 minutes more.
7.Mix the remaining oil mixture with rosemary and breadcrumbs in a bowl.
8.Spread this mixture over the Brussels sprouts and return the basket to the fryer.
9.Air fry them for 5 minutes.
10. Enjoy.

Nutrition

Calories: 246 kcal/Cal
Fat: 7.4 g
Carbohydrates: 9.4 g
Fiber: 2.7 g
Protein: 37.2 g

59.Peach-Bourbon Wings

Preparation Time: 5 minutes
Cooking Time: 14 minutes
Servings: 8

Ingredients

- ½ cup peach preserves
- 1 tbsp. brown sugar
- 1 garlic clove, minced

- ¼ tsp. salt
- 1 tbsp. white vinegar
- 1 tbsp. bourbon
- 1 tsp. cornstarch
- 1½ tsp. water
- lbs. chicken wings

Directions

1.Let your air fryer preheat at 400°F.
2.Add salt, garlic, and brown sugar to a food processor and blend well until smooth.
3.Transfer this mixture to a saucepan and add bourbon, peach preserves, and vinegar.
4.Cook this mixture to a boil, then reduce heat to a simmer.
5.Cook for 6 minutes until the mixture thickens.
6.Mix cornstarch with water and pour this mixture into the saucepan.
7.Cook for 2 minutes until it thickens. Keep ¼ cup of this sauce aside.
8.Place the wings in the air fryer basket and brush them with prepared sauce.
9.Return the fryer basket to the air fryer and cook on air fry mode for 6 minutes at 350°F.
10. Flip the wings and brush them again with the sauce.
11. Air fry the wings for another 8 minutes.
12. Serve with reserved sauce.

Nutrition

Calories: 293 kcal/Cal
Fat: 16 g
Carbohydrates: 5.2 g
Fiber: 1.9 g
Protein: 34.2 g

60.Reuben Calzones

Preparation Time: 5 minutes
Cooking Time: 12 minutes
Servings: 4
Ingredients

- 1 tube (13.8 ounces) refrigerated pizza crust
- slices Swiss cheese
- 1 cup sauerkraut, rinsed and well drained
- ½ lb. corned beef, sliced & cooked

Directions

1.Let your air fryer preheat at 400°F. Grease the air fryer basket with cooking oil.
2.Spread the pizza crust on a lightly floured surface into a 12-inch square.
3.Slice the crust into four smaller squares.
4.Place one slice of cheese, ¼ of the sauerkraut, and 1 slice of corned beef over each square diagonally.
5.Fold the squares in half diagonally to form a triangle and pinch the edges together.
6.Place 2 triangles in the air fryer basket at a time and spray them with cooking oil.
7.Return the fryer basket to the air fryer and cook on air fry mode for 12 minutes at 350°F.
8.Air fry the remaining calzone triangles.
9.Enjoy with fresh salad.

Nutrition

Calories: 604 kcal/Cal
Fat: 30.6 g
Carbohydrates: 31.4 g
Fiber: 0.2 g
Protein: 54.6 g

61.Braised Pork

Preparation Time: 40 minutes
Cooking Time: 40 minutes
Servings: 2
Ingredients

- 1-pound pork loin roast, boneless and cubed
- 2 tablespoons butter, melted and divided
- Salt and black pepper, to taste
- 1 cup chicken stock
- ¼ cup dry white wine
- 1 clove garlic, minced
- ½ teaspoon thyme, chopped
- ½ thyme sprig
- 1 bay leaf
- ¼ yellow onion, chopped
- 1 tablespoon white flour
- ¼ pound red grapes

Directions

1.Season pork cubes with salt and pepper. Rub with half the melted butter and put in the air fryer. Cook at 370F for 8 minutes.
2.Meanwhile, heat a pan on the stove with 2 tablespoons of butter over medium heat. Add onion and garlic, and stir-fry for 2 minutes.
3.Add bay leaf, flour, thyme, salt, pepper, stock, and wine. Mix well. Bring to a simmer and take off the heat.
4.Add grapes and pork cubes. Cook in the air fryer at 360°F for 30 minutes.
5.Serve.

Nutrition
Calories: 320 kcal/Cal
Fat: 4 g
Carbohydrates: 29 g
Protein: 38 g

62.Lean Beef with Green Onions

Preparation Time: 10 minutes
Cooking Time: 20 minutes
Servings: 2
Ingredients

- ½ cup green onion, chopped
- ½ cup soy sauce
- ¼ cup water
- 2 tablespoons brown sugar
- 2 tablespoons sesame seeds
- cloves garlic, minced
- ½ teaspoon black pepper
- ½ pound lean beef

Directions
1.In a bowl, mix the onion with water, soy sauce, garlic, sugar, sesame seeds, and pepper. Whisk and add meat. Marinate for 10 minutes.
2.Drain beef. Preheat the air fryer to 390F, then cook beef for 20 minutes.
3.Serve.

Nutrition
Calories: 329 kcal/Cal
Fat: 8 g
Carbohydrates: 26 g
Protein: 22 g

Chapter 9.Dinner

63.Sweet & Spicy Country-Style Ribs

Preparation Time: 10 minutes
Cooking Time: 25 minutes
Servings: 4
Ingredients:

- 2 tablespoons brown sugar
- 2 tablespoons smoked paprika
- 1 teaspoon garlic powder
- 1 teaspoon onion powder
- 1 teaspoon dry mustard
- 1 teaspoon ground cumin
- 1 teaspoon kosher salt
- 1 teaspoon black pepper
- ¼ to ½ teaspoon cayenne pepper
- 1½ pounds boneless country-style pork ribs
- 1 cup barbecue sauce

Directions:

1.Preparing the Ingredients. In a small bowl, stir together the brown sugar, paprika, garlic powder, onion powder, dry mustard, cumin, salt, black pepper, and cayenne. Mix until well combined.
2.Pat the ribs dry with a paper towel. Generously sprinkle the rub evenly over both sides of the ribs and rub in with your fingers.
3.Air Frying. Place the ribs in the air fryer basket. Set the Pro Breeze air fryer to 350°F for 15 minutes.
4.Turn the ribs and brush with ½ cup of the barbecue sauce. Cook for an additional 10 minutes. Use a meat thermometer to ensure the pork has reached an internal temperature of 145°F.
5.Serve with remaining barbecue sauce.

Nutrition:

Calories: 416 kcal
Protein: 38.39 g
Fat: 12.19 g
Carbohydrates: 36.79 g

64.Pork Tenders with Bell Peppers

Preparation Time: 5 minutes
Cooking Time: 15 minutes
Servings: 4
Ingredients:

- Oz Pork Tenderloin
- 1 Bell Pepper, in thin strips
- 1 Red Onion, sliced
- 1 Tsps. Provencal Herbs
- Black Pepper to taste
- 1 tbsp. Olive Oil
- 1/2 tbsp. Mustard

Directions:

1.Preparing the Ingredients. Preheat the Pro Breeze air fryer to 390 degrees.
2.In the oven dish, mix the bell pepper strips with the onion, herbs, and some salt and pepper to taste.
3.Add half a tablespoon of olive oil to the mixture
4.Cut the pork tenderloin into four pieces and rub with salt, pepper, and mustard.
5.Thinly coat the pieces with remaining olive oil and place them upright in the oven dish on top of the pepper mixture
6.Air Frying. Place the bowl into the air fryer. Set the timer to 15 minutes and roast the meat and the vegetables
7.Turn the meat and mix the peppers halfway through
8.Serve with a fresh salad

Nutrition:

Calories: 220 kcal
Protein: 23.79 g
Fat: 12.36 g
Carbohydrates: 2.45 g

65.Wonton Meatballs

Preparation Time: 15 minutes
Cooking Time: 10 minutes
Servings: 4
Ingredients:

- 1-pound ground pork
- large eggs
- ¼ cup chopped green onions (white and green parts)
- ¼ cup chopped fresh cilantro or parsley
- 1 tablespoon minced fresh ginger
- cloves garlic, minced
- 1 teaspoons soy sauce
- 1 teaspoon oyster sauce
- ½ teaspoon kosher salt
- 1 teaspoon black pepper

Directions:

1.Preparing the Ingredients. In the bowl of a stand mixer fitted with the paddle attachment, combine the pork, eggs, green onions, cilantro, ginger, garlic, soy sauce, oyster sauce, salt, and pepper. Mix on low speed until all of the ingredients are incorporated, 2 to 3 minutes.
2.Form the mixture into 12 meatballs and arrange in a single layer in the air fryer basket.
3.Air Frying. Set the Pro Breeze air fryer to 350°F for 10 minutes. Use a meat thermometer to ensure the meatballs have reached an internal temperature of 145°F.
4.Transfer the meatballs to a bowl and serve.
Nutrition:
Calories: 402 kcal
Protein: 32.69 g
Fat: 27.91 g
Carbohydrates: 3.1 g

66.Barbecue Flavored Pork Ribs

Preparation Time: 5 minutes
Cooking Time:15 minutes
Servings: 6
Ingredients:

- ¼ cup honey, divided
- ¾ cup BBQ sauce
- 2 tablespoons tomato ketchup
- 1 tablespoon Worcestershire sauce
- 1 tablespoon soy sauce
- ½ teaspoon garlic powder
- Freshly ground white pepper to taste
- 1¾ pound pork ribs

Directions:
1.Preparing the Ingredients. In a large bowl, mix together 3 tablespoons of honey and remaining ingredients except for pork ribs. Refrigerate to marinate for about 20 minutes. Preheat the Pro Breeze air fryer to 355 degrees F. Place the ribs in an Air fryer basket.
2.Air Frying. Cook for about 13 minutes. Remove the ribs from the Air fryer and coat with remaining honey.
3.Serve hot.
Nutrition:
Calories: 265 kcal
Protein: 29.47 g
Fat: 9.04 g
Carbohydrates: 15.87 g

67.Easy Air Fryer Marinated Pork Tenderloin

Preparation Time: 1 hour & 10 minutes
Cooking Time: 30 minutes
Servings: 4 to 6
Ingredients:

- ¼ cup olive oil
- ¼ cup soy sauce
- ¼ cup freshly squeezed lemon juice
- 1 garlic clove, minced
- 1 tablespoon Dijon mustard
- 1 teaspoon salt
- ½ teaspoon freshly ground black pepper
- pounds pork tenderloin

Directions:
1.Preparing the Ingredients. In a large mixing bowl, make the marinade. Mix together the olive oil, soy sauce, lemon juice, minced garlic, Dijon mustard, salt, and pepper. Reserve ¼ cup of the marinade.
2.Place the tenderloin in a large bowl and pour the remaining marinade over the meat. Cover and marinate in the refrigerator for about 1 hour. Place the marinated pork tenderloin into the air fryer basket.
3.Air Frying. Set the temperature of your Pro Breeze AF to 400°F. Set the timer and roast for 10 minutes. Using tongs, flip the pork and baste it with half of the reserved marinade. Reset the timer and roast for 10 minutes more.
4.Using tongs, flip the pork, then baste with the remaining marinade.
5.Reset the timer and roast for another 10 minutes for a total cooking time of 30 minutes.
Nutrition:
Calories: 345 kcal
Protein: 41.56 g
Fat: 17.35 g
Carbohydrates: 3.66 g

68.Balsamic Glazed Pork Chops

Preparation Time: 5 minutes
Cooking Time: 50
Servings: 4
Ingredients:

- ¾ cup balsamic vinegar
- 1 ½ tablespoons sugar

- 1 tablespoon butter
- 2 tablespoons olive oil
- 2 tablespoons salt
- pork rib chops

Directions:

1.Preparing the Ingredients. Place all ingredients in a bowl and allow the meat to marinate in the fridge for at least 2 hours. Preheat the Pro Breeze air fryer to 390°F. Place the grill pan accessory in the air fryer.
2.Air Frying. Grill the pork chops for 20 minutes, making sure to flip the meat every 10 minutes for even grilling. Meanwhile, pour the balsamic vinegar into a saucepan and allow to simmer for at least 10 minutes until the sauce thickens.
3.Brush the meat with the glaze before serving.

Nutrition:

Calories: 274
Fat: 18g
Protein:17g

69.Perfect Air Fried Pork Chops

Preparation Time: 5 minutes
Cooking Time: 17 minutes
Servings: 4
Ingredients:

- 2 cups bread crumbs
- ½ cup grated Parmesan cheese
- 2 tablespoons vegetable oil
- 2 teaspoons salt
- 2 teaspoons sweet paprika
- ½ teaspoon onion powder
- ¼ teaspoon garlic powder
- (½-inch-thick) bone-in pork chops

Directions:

1.Preparing the Ingredients. Spray the Pro Breeze air fryer basket with olive oil. In a large resealable bag, combine the bread crumbs, Parmesan cheese, oil, salt, paprika, onion powder, and garlic powder. Seal the bag and shake it a few times in order for the spices to blend together. Place the pork chops, one by one, in the bag, and shake to coat.
2.Air Frying. Place the pork chops in the greased Pro Breeze air fryer basket in a single layer. Be careful not to overcrowd the basket. Spray the chops generously with olive oil to avoid powdery, uncooked breading.
3.Set the temperature of your Pro Breeze AF to 360°F. Set the timer and roast for 10 minutes.
4.Using tongs, flip the chops. Spray them generously with olive oil.
5.Reset the timer and roast for 7 minutes more.
6.Check that the pork has reached an internal temperature of 145°F. Add cooking time if needed.

Nutrition:

Calories: 513
Fat: 23g
Saturated fat: 8g
Carbohydrate: 22g
Fiber: 2g
Sugar: 3g
Protein: 50g
Iron: 3mg;
Sodium: 1521mg

70.Rustic Pork Ribs

Preparation Time: 5 minutes
Cooking Time: 15 minutes
Servings: 4
Ingredients:

- 1 rack of pork ribs
- 2 tablespoons dry red wine
- 1 tablespoon soy sauce
- 1/2 teaspoon dried thyme
- 1/2 teaspoon onion powder
- 1/2 teaspoon garlic powder
- 1/2 teaspoon ground black pepper
- 1 teaspoon smoke salt
- 1 tablespoon cornstarch
- 1/2 teaspoon olive oil

Directions:

1.Preparing the Ingredients. Begin by preheating your Air fryer to 390 degrees F. Place all ingredients in a mixing bowl and let them marinate at least 1 hour.
2.Air Frying. Cook the marinated ribs for approximately 25 minutes at 390 degrees F.
3.Serve hot.

Nutrition:

Calories: 119 kcal
Protein: 12.26 g
Fat: 5.61 g

Carbohydrates: 3.64 g

71.Air Fryer Baby Back Ribs

Preparation Time: 5 minutes
Cooking Time: 25 minutes
Servings: 4
Ingredients:

- 1 rack baby back ribs
- 1 tablespoon garlic powder
- 1 teaspoon freshly ground black pepper
- 2 tablespoons salt
- 1 cup barbecue sauce (any type)

Directions:

1.Preparing the Ingredients
2.Dry the ribs with a paper towel.
3.Season the ribs with the garlic powder, pepper, and salt.
4.Place the seasoned ribs into the air fryer.
5.Air Frying.
6.Set the temperature of your Pro Breeze AF to 400°F. Set the timer and grill for 10 minutes.
7.Using tongs, flip the ribs.
8.Reset the timer and grill for another 10 minutes.
9.Once the ribs are cooked, use a pastry brush to brush on the barbecue sauce, then set the timer and grill for a final 3 to 5 minutes.

Nutrition:

Calories: 422
Fat: 27g
Saturated fat: 10g
Carbohydrate: 25g
Fiber: 1g
Sugar: 17g
Protein: 18g
Iron: 1mg
Sodium: 4273mg

72.Parmesan Crusted Pork Chops

Preparation Time: 10 minutes
Cooking Time: 15 minutes
Servings: 8
Ingredients:

- 1 tbsp. grated parmesan cheese
- 1 C. pork rind crumbs
- 4 beaten eggs
- ¼ tsp. chili powder
- ½ tsp. onion powder
- 1 tsp. smoked paprika
- ¼ tsp. pepper
- ½ tsp. salt
- 4-6 thick boneless pork chops

Directions:

1.Preparing the Ingredients. Ensure your air fryer is preheated to 400 degrees.
2.With pepper and salt, season both sides of pork chops.
3.In a food processor, pulse pork rinds into crumbs. Mix crumbs with other seasonings.
4.Beat eggs and add to another bowl.
5.Dip pork chops into eggs then into pork rind crumb mixture.
6.Air Frying. Spray down air fryer with olive oil and add pork chops to the basket. Set temperature to 400°F, and set time to 15 minutes.

Nutrition:

Calories: 422
Fat: 19g
Protein:38g
Sugar:2g

73.Crispy Dumplings

Preparation Time: 10 minutes
Cooking Time: 10 minutes
Servings: 8
Ingredients:

- .5 lb. Ground pork
- 1 tbsp. Olive oil
- .5 tsp each Black pepper and salt
- Half of 1 pkg. Dumpling wrappers

Directions:

1.Set the Air Fryer temperature setting at 390º Fahrenheit.
2.Mix the fixings together.
3.Prepare each dumpling using two teaspoons of the pork mixture.
4.Seal the edges with a portion of water to make the triangle form.

5.Lightly spritz the Air Fryer basket using a cooking oil spray as needed. Add the dumplings to air-fry for eight minutes.
6.Serve when they're ready.

Nutrition:

Calories: 110 kcal
Protein: 8.14 g
Fat: 8.34 g
Carbohydrates: 0.27 g

74.Pork Joint

Preparation Time: 10 minutes
Cooking Time: 20 minutes
Servings: 10

Ingredients:

- 2 cups Cooked shredded pork tenderloin or chicken
- 2 cups Fat-free shredded mozzarella
- small Flour tortillas
- Lime juice

Directions:

1.Set the Air Fryer at 380º Fahrenheit.
2.Sprinkle the juice over the pork.
3.Microwave five of the tortillas at a time (putting a damp paper towel over them for 10 seconds). Add three ounces of pork and ¼ of a cup of cheese to each tortilla.
4.Tightly roll the tortillas. Line the tortillas into a greased foil-lined pan.
5.Spray an even coat of cooking oil spray over the tortillas.
6.Air Fry for 7 to 10 minutes or until the tortillas are a golden color, flipping halfway through.

Nutrition:

Calories: 334 kcal
Protein: 32.03 g
Fat: 6.87 g
Carbohydrates: 33.92 g

Chapter 10.Dinner 2

75.Mouthwatering Shredded BBQ Roast

Preparation Time: 10 minutes
Cooking Time: 30 minutes
Servings: 8
Ingredients:

- lbs. pork roast
- 1 tsp. garlic powder
- Salt and pepper to taste
- 1/2 cup water
- can (11 oz.) of barbecue sauce, keno unsweetened

Directions:

1.Season the pork with garlic powder, salt, and pepper, place in your Breville smart air fryer.
2.Pour water and lock lid into place; set on the MEAT/STEW, high-pressure setting for 30 minutes.
3.When ready, use Quick Release - turn the valve from sealing to venting to release the pressure.
4.Remove pork in a bowl, and with two forks, shred the meat.
5.Pour BBQ sauce and stir to combine well.
6.Serve.

Nutrition:
Calories: 373 kcal/Cal
Carbohydrates: 2.5 g
Proteins: 34 g
Fat: 24 g
Fiber: 3 g

76.Sour and Spicy Spareribs

Preparation Time: 15 minutes
Cooking Time: 35 minutes
Servings: 10
Ingredients

- lbs. spare spareribs
- Salt and pepper to taste
- 1 Tbsp. of tallow
- 1/2 cup coconut amines (from coconut sap)
- 1/2 cup vinegar
- 1 Tbsp. Worcestershire sauce to taste
- 1 tsp. chili powder
- 1 tsp. garlic powder
- 1 tsp. celery seeds

Directions:

1. Cut the rack of ribs into equal portions.
2. Season with salt and ground pepper your spareribs from all sides.
3. Add tallow in your Breville smart air fryer and place spareribs.
4. In a bowl, combine all remaining ingredients and pour over spareribs.
5. Lock lid into place and set on the MANUAL setting on HIGH heat for 35 minutes.
6. When the timer beeps, press "Cancel" and carefully flip the Natural Release for 20 minutes.
7. Open the lid and transfer ribs on a serving platter.
8. Serve hot.

Nutrition:
Calories: 598 kcal/Cal
Carbohydrates: 2 g
Proteins: 36 g
Fat: 54 g
Fiber: 0.2 g

77.Tender Pork Shoulder with Hot Peppers

Preparation Time: 10 minutes
Cooking Time: 30 minutes
Servings: 8
Ingredients:

- lbs. pork shoulder boneless
- Salt and ground black pepper to taste
- 1 Tbsp. of olive oil
- 1 large onion, chopped
- cloves garlic minced
- \- 3 chili peppers, chopped
- 1 tsp. ground coriander
- 1 tsp. ground cumin
- 1 ½ cups of bone broth (preferably homemade)
- 1/2 cup water

Directions:

1.Season with salt and pepper the pork meat.
2.Turn on the Breville smart air fryer and press the SAUTÉ button. When the word "hot" appears on display, add the oil and

sauté the onions and garlic for about 5 minutes.
3.Add pork and sear for 1 - 2 minutes from all sides; turn off the SAUTÉ button.
4.Add all remaining ingredients into Breville smart air fryer.
5.Lock lid into place and set on the MEAT/STEW setting on HIGH heat for 30 minutes.
6.When the timer beeps, press "Cancel" and carefully flip the Natural Release button for 15 minutes.
7.Serve hot.
Nutrition:
Calories: 389 kcal/Cal
Carbohydrates: 2.5 g
Proteins: 36 g
Fat: 27 g
Fiber: 0.5 g

78.Braised Sour Pork Filet

Preparation Time: 10 minutes
Cooking Time: 8 hours
Servings: 6
Ingredients:

- 1/2 tsp. of dry thyme
- 1/2 tsp. of sage
- Salt and ground black pepper to taste
- Tabs of olive oil
- lbs. of pork fillet
- 1/3 cup of shallots (chopped)
- cloves of garlic (minced)
- 3/4 cup of bone broth
- 1/3 cup of apple cider vinegar

Directions:
1.In a small bowl, combine thyme, sage, salt, and black ground pepper.
2.Rub generously pork from all sides.
3.Heat the olive oil in a large frying pan, and sear pork for 2 - 3 minutes.
4.Place pork in your Crock Pot and add shallots and garlic.
5.Pour broth and apple cider vinegar/juice.
6.Cover and cook on SLOW for 8 hours or on HIGH for 4-5 hours.
7.Remove pork on a plate, adjust salt and pepper, slice, and serve with cooking juice.
Nutrition:
Calories: 348 kcal/Cal
Carbohydrates: 3 g
Proteins: 51 g
Fat: 12.5 g
Fiber: 0.1 g

79.Pork with Anise and Cumin Stir-fry

Preparation Time: 5 minutes
Cooking Time: 30 minutes
Servings: 4
Ingredients:

- 1 Tbsp. lard
- spring onions finely chopped (only green part)
- cloves garlic, finely chopped
- 2 lbs. pork loin, boneless, cut into cubes
- Sea salt and black ground pepper to taste
- 1 green bell pepper (cut into thin strips)
- 1/2 cup water
- 1/2 tsp. dill seeds
- 1/2 anise seeds
- 1/2 tsp. cumin

Directions:

1. Heat the lard n a large frying pot over medium-high heat.
2. Sauté the spring onions and garlic with a pinch of salt for 3 - 4 minutes.
3. Add the pork and simmer for about 5 - 6 minutes.
4. Add all remaining ingredients and stir well.
5. Cover and let simmer for 15 - 20 minutes
6. Taste and adjust seasoning to taste.
7. Serve!

Nutrition:
Calories: 351 kcal/Cal
Carbohydrates: 3 g
Proteins: 1 g
Fat: 51.5 g
Fiber: 1 g

80.Baked Meatballs with Goat Cheese

Preparation Time: 15 minutes
Cooking Time: 35 minutes
Servings: 8
Ingredients:

- 1 Tbsp. of tallow
- lbs. of ground beef

- 1 organic egg
- 1 grated onion
- 1/2 cup of almond milk (unsweetened)
- 1 cup of red wine
- 1/2 bunch of chopped parsley
- 1/2 cup of almond flour
- Salt and ground pepper to taste
- 1/2 Tbsp. of dry oregano
- oz. of hard goat cheese cut in cubes

Directions:

1.Preheat oven to 400°F.
2.Grease a baking pan with tallow.
3.In a large bowl, combine all ingredients except goat cheese.
4.Knead the mixture until ingredients are evenly combined.
5.Make small meatballs and place in a prepared baking dish.
6.Place one cube of cheese on each meatball.
7.Bake for 30 - 35 minutes.
8.Serve hot.

Nutrition:

Calories: 404 kcal/Cal
Carbohydrates: 2.2 g
Proteins: 25.5 g
Fat: 31 g
Fiber: 0.5 g

81.Parisian Schnitzel

Preparation Time: 15 minutes
Cooking Time: 10 minutes
Servings: 4
Ingredients:

- veal steaks; thin schnitzel
- Salt and ground black pepper
- 1 Tbsp. of butter
- 4 eggs from free-range chickens
- 1 Tbsp. of almond flour

Directions:

1.Season steaks with salt and pepper.
2.Heat butter in a large nonstick frying pan at medium heat.
3.In a bowl, beat the eggs.
4.Add almond flour in a bowl.
5.Roll each steak in almond flour, add then, dip in beaten eggs.
6.Fry about 3 minutes per side.
7.Serve right away.

Nutrition:

Calories: 355 kcal/Cal
Carbohydrates: 0.3 g
Proteins: 54 g
Fat: 15 g
Fiber: 0 g

82.Keto Beef Stroganoff

Preparation Time: 5 minutes
Cooking Time: 30 minutes
Servings: 6
Ingredients:

- lbs. of rump or round steak or stewing steak
- 1 Tbsp. of olive oil
- green onions, finely chopped
- 1 grated tomato
- 1 Tbsp. ketchup (without sugar)
- 1 cup of button mushrooms
- 1/2 cup of bone broth
- 1 cup of sour cream
- Salt and black pepper to taste

Directions:

1. Cut the meat into strips and sauté in a large frying skillet.
2. Add chopped onion and a pinch of salt and cook meat for about 20 minutes at medium temperature.
3. Add mushrooms and ketchup and stir for 3 - 5 minutes.
4. Pour the bone broth and sour cream and cook for 3 - 4 minutes.
5. Remove from the heat, taste, and adjust salt and pepper to taste.
6. Serve hot.

Nutrition:

Calories: 348 kcal/Cal
Carbohydrates: 4.2 g
Proteins: 37 g
Fat: 21 g
Fiber: 1 g

83.Meatloaf with Gruyere

Preparation Time: 15 minutes
Cooking Time: 40 minutes
Servings: 6
Ingredients:

- 1 1/2 lbs. ground beef
- 1 cup ground almonds
- 1 large egg from free-range chickens
- 1/2 cup grated Gruyere cheese
- 1 tsp. fresh parsley finely chopped
- 1 scallion finely chopped

- 1/2 tsp. ground cumin
- 4 eggs boiled
- 1 Tbsp. of fresh grass-fed butter, melted

Directions:

1.Preheat oven to 350°F.
2.Combine all ingredients (except eggs and butter) in a large bowl.
3.Using your hands, combine the mixture well.
4.Shape the mixture into a roll and place in the middle sliced hard-boiled eggs.
5.Transfer the meatloaf to a 5x9 inch loaf pan greased with melted butter.
6.Place in oven and bake for 40 minutes or until an internal temperature of 160°F.
7.Remove from the oven and allow rest for 10 minutes.
8.Slice and serve.

Nutrition:

Calories: 598 kcal/Cal
Carbohydrates: 5.3 g
Proteins: 28 g
Fat: 63 g
Fiber: 2.6 g

84.Roasted Filet Mignon in Foil

Preparation Time: 15 minutes
Cooking Time: 45 minutes
Servings: 8
Ingredients:

- lbs. filet mignon in one piece
- Salt to taste and ground black pepper
- 1 tsp. of garlic powder
- 1 tsp. of onion powder
- 1 tsp. of cumin
- 1 Tbsp. of olive oil

Directions:

1.Preheat the oven to 425°F.
2.Rinse and clean the filet mignon, removing all fats, or ask your butcher to do it for you.
3.Season with salt and pepper, garlic powder, onion powder, and cumin.
4.Wrap filet mignon in foil and place in a roasting pan, drizzle with the olive oil.
5.Roast for 15 minutes per pound for medium-rare or to desired doneness.
6.Remove from the oven and allow to rest for 10 -15 minutes before serving.

Nutrition:

Calories: 350 kcal/Cal
Carbohydrates: 0.8 g
Proteins: 52.5 g
Fat: 12.2 g
Fiber: 0.2 g

85.Stewed Beef with Green Beans

Preparation Time: 10 minutes
Cooking Time: 50 minutes
Servings: 8
Ingredients:

- 1/2 cup olive oil
- 1 1/2 lbs. beef cut into cubes
- scallions, finely chopped
- 4 cups water
- 1 lb. fresh green beans - trimmed and cut diagonally in half
- 1 bay leaf
- 1 grated tomato
- 1/2 cup fresh mint leaves, finely chopped
- 1 tsp. fresh or dry rosemary
- Salt and freshly ground pepper to taste

Directions:

1. Chop the beef into 1-inch thick cubes.
2. Heat the olive oil in a large pot at high heat. Sauté the beef for about 4 - 5 minutes, sprinkle with a pinch of salt and pepper.
3. Add the scallions and stir and sauté for about another 3 - 4 minutes until softened. Pour water and cook for 2-3 minutes.
4. Add the bay leaf and grated tomato. Cook for about 5 minutes; lower the heat at medium-low. Cover and simmer for about 15 minutes.
5. Add the green beans, rosemary, salt, fresh ground pepper, and water enough to cover all ingredients. Gently simmer for 15 - 20 minutes until the green beans are tender.
6. Sprinkle with the mint and rosemary, gently mix and remove from the heat. Serve hot.

Nutrition:

Calories: 354 kcal/Cal
Carbohydrates: 6 g
Proteins: 23 g
Fat: 26.5 g
Fiber: 2.7 g

86.Turkey and Quinoa Stuffed Peppers

Preparation Time: 15 minutes
Cooking Time: 35 minutes
Servings: 6
Ingredients:

- large red bell peppers
- 1 tsp. chopped fresh rosemary
- 1 tbsp. chopped fresh parsley
- 1 tbsp. chopped pecans, toasted
- 1 tbsp. extra virgin olive oil
- ½ cup chicken stock
- ½ lb. fully cooked smoked turkey sausage, diced
- ½ tsp. salt
- 2 cups water
- 1 cup uncooked quinoa

Directions:

1.On high fire, place a large saucepan and add salt, water, and quinoa. Bring to a boil.
2.Once boiling, reduce fire to a simmer, cover, and cook until all water is absorbed, around 15 minutes.
3.Uncover quinoa, turn off the fire, and let it stand for another 5 minutes.
4.Slice peppers lengthwise in half and discard membranes and seeds. In another boiling pot of water, add peppers, boil for 5 minutes, drain and discard water.
5.Grease a 13 x 9 baking dish and preheat oven to 350oF.
6.Place boiled bell pepper onto a prepared baking dish, evenly fill with the quinoa mixture, and pop into the oven.
7.Bake for 15 minutes.

Nutrition:

Calories: 253 kcal/Cal
Total Fat: 13 g
Saturated Fat: 2 g
Total Carbs: 21 g
Net Carbs: 19.7 g
Protein: 14 g
Sugar: 1.3 g
Fiber: 3 g
Sodium: 545 mg
Potassium: 372 mg

Chapter 11.Mains

87.Succulent Turkey Cakes

Preparation Time: 10 minutes
Cooking Time: 20 Minutes
Servings: 4
Ingredients:

- mushrooms; chopped
- 1 tsp. garlic powder
- 1 tsp. onion powder
- 1 ¼ lbs. turkey meat; ground
- Cooking spray
- Tomato sauce for serving
- Salt and black pepper to the taste

Directions:
1.In your blender, mix mushrooms with salt and pepper, pulse well and transfer to a bowl.
2.Add turkey, onion powder, garlic powder, salt, and pepper; stir and shape cakes out of this mix.
3.Spray them with cooking spray; transfer them to your air fryer and cook at 320 °F for 10 minutes. Serve them with tomato sauce on the side and a tasty side salad.
Nutrition:
Calories: 202;
Fat: 6;
Fiber: 3;
Carbs: 17;
Protein: 10

88.Potato Salad

Preparation Time: 10 minutes
Cooking Time: 35 Minutes
Servings: 4
Ingredients:

- lb. red potatoes; halved
- 1 tbsp. olive oil
- 1/3 cup lemon juice
- 1 tbsp. mustard
- Salt and black pepper to the taste
- green onions; chopped
- 1 red bell pepper; chopped

Directions:
1. On your air fryer's basket, mix potatoes with half of the olive oil, salt, and pepper and cook at 350 °F for 25 minutes, shaking the fryer once.
2. In a bowl, mix onions with bell pepper and roasted potatoes and toss.
3. In a small bowl, mix lemon juice with the rest of the oil and mustard and whisk really well. Add this to potato salad; toss well and serve for lunch.
Nutrition:
Calories: 211;
Fat: 6;
Fiber: 8;
Carbs: 12;
Protein: 4

89.Buttermilk Chicken

Preparation Time: 10 minutes
Cooking Time: 28 Minutes
Servings: 4
Ingredients:

- 1 ½ lbs. chicken thighs
- 2 cups buttermilk
- 1 tbsp. baking powder
- 1 tbsp. sweet paprika
- A pinch of cayenne pepper
- 2 cups white flour
- 1 tbsp. garlic powder
- Salt and black pepper to the taste

Directions:
1.In a bowl, mix chicken thighs with buttermilk, salt, pepper, and cayenne; toss and leave aside for 6 hours.
2.In a separate bowl, mix flour with paprika, baking powder, and garlic powder and stir.
3.Drain chicken thighs, dredge them in the flour mix, arrange them in your air fryer and cook at 360 °F for 8 minutes. Flip chicken pieces, cook them for 10 minutes more, arrange on a platter, and serve for lunch.
Nutrition:
Calories: 200;
Fat: 3;
Fiber: 9;
Carbs: 14;
Protein: 4

90.Cheese Burgers

Preparation Time: 10 minutes
Cooking Time: 30 Minutes
Servings: 2
Ingredients:

- oz. lean beef; ground
- 1 tsp. ketchup

- 1 tbsp. yellow onion; chopped.
- 1 tsp. mustard
- cheddar cheese slices
- burger buns; halved
- Salt and black pepper to the taste

Directions:

1.In a bowl, mix beef with onion, ketchup, mustard, salt, and pepper; stir well and shape 4 patties out of this mix.

2.Divide cheese into 2 patties and top with the other 2 patties.

3.Place them in a preheated air fryer at 370 °F and fry them for 20 minutes. Divide cheeseburger into 2 bun halves; top with the other 2 serve for lunch.

Nutrition:

Calories: 261;
Fat: 6;
Fiber: 10;
Carbs: 20;
Protein: 6

91.Creamy Chicken Stew Recipe

Preparation Time: 10 minutes
Cooking Time: 35 Minutes
Servings: 4
Ingredients:

- 1 ½ cups canned cream of celery soup
- chicken tenders
- 1 tbsp. milk
- 1 egg yolk
- 1/2 cup heavy cream
- potatoes; chopped
- 1 bay leaf
- 1 thyme spring; chopped
- Salt and black pepper to the taste

Directions:

1.In a bowl, mix chicken with cream of celery, potatoes, heavy cream, bay leaf, thyme, salt, and pepper; toss, pour into your air fryer's pan, and cook at 320 °F, for 25 minutes.

2.Leave your stew to cool down a bit; discard bay leaf, divide among plates, and serve right away.

Nutrition:

Calories: 300;
Fat: 11;
Fiber: 2;
Carbs: 23;
Protein: 14

92.Tasty Hot Dogs

Preparation Time: 10 minutes
Cooking Time: 17 Minutes
Servings: 2
Ingredients:

- hot dog buns
- 1 tbsp. Dijon mustard
- hot dogs
- 1 tbsp. cheddar cheese; grated

Directions:

1. Put hot dogs in preheated air fryer and cook them at 390 °F for 5 minutes.
2. Divide hot dogs into hot dog buns, spread mustard and cheese; return everything to your air fryer and cook for 2 minutes more at 390 degrees F. Serve for lunch.

Nutrition:

Calories: 211;
Fat: 3;
Fiber: 8;
Carbs: 12;
Protein: 4

93.Chicken Corn Casserole

Preparation Time: 10 minutes
Cooking Time: 40 Minutes
Servings: 6
Ingredients:

- 1 cup clean chicken stock
- oz. canned coconut milk
- 1 ½ cups green lentils
- lbs. chicken breasts; skinless, boneless, and cubed
- 1/3 cup cilantro; chopped
- 2 cups corn
- handfuls spinach
- green onions; chopped
- 1 tsp. garlic powder
- Salt and black pepper to the taste

Directions:

1.In a pan that fits your air fryer, mix stock with coconut milk, salt, pepper, garlic powder, chicken, and lentils.

2.Add corn, green onions, cilantro, and spinach; stir well,

3. introduce in your air fryer and cook at 350 °F for 30 minutes.

Nutrition:

Calories: 345;

Fat: 12;
Fiber: 10;
Carbs: 20;
Protein: 44

94.Veggie Toasts

Preparation Time: 10 minutes
Cooking Time: 25 Minutes
Servings: 4
Ingredients:

- 1 red bell pepper; cut into thin strips
- 1 cup cremini mushrooms; sliced
- bread slices
- 1 tbsp. butter; soft
- 1 yellow squash; chopped.
- green onions; sliced
- 1 tbsp. olive oil
- 1/2 cup goat cheese; crumbled

Directions:
1.In a bowl, mix red bell pepper with mushrooms, squash, green onions, and oil, toss; transfer to your air fryer, cook them at 350 °F, for 10 minutes; shaking the fryer once and transfer them to a bowl.
2.Spread butter on bread slices; place them in the air fryer and cook them at 350 °F for 5 minutes. Divide veggie mix on each bread slice, top with crumbled cheese, and serve for lunch.
Nutrition:
Calories: 152;
Fat: 3;
Fiber: 4;
Carbs: 7;
Protein: 2

95.Succulent Turkey Breast

Preparation Time: 10 minutes
Cooking Time: 57 Minutes
Servings: 4
Ingredients:

- 1 big turkey breast
- 1 tsp. olive oil
- 1/2 tsp. smoked paprika
- 1 tsp. thyme; dried
- 1/2 tsp. sage; dried
- 1 tbsp. mustard
- 1/4 cup maple syrup
- 1 tbsp. butter; soft
- Salt and black pepper to the taste

Directions:
1.Brush turkey breast with the olive oil; season with salt, pepper, thyme, paprika, and sage, rub, place in your air fryer's basket and fry at 350 °F, for 25 minutes.
2.Flip turkey; cook for 10 minutes more; flip one more time and cook for another 10 minutes.
3.Meanwhile, heat up a pan with the butter over medium heat, add mustard and maple syrup, stir well, cook for a couple of minutes and take off the heat. Slice turkey breast, divide among plates, and serve with the maple glaze drizzled on top.
Nutrition:
Calories: 280;
Fat: 2;
Fiber: 7;
Carbs: 16;
Protein: 14

96.Bell Pepper and Sausage

Preparation Time: 10 minutes
Cooking Time: 20 Minutes
Servings: 4
Ingredients:

- 1 lb. sausages; sliced
- 1 red bell pepper; cut into strips
- 1/2 cup yellow onion; chopped.
- 1/2 cup chicken stock
- 1/3 cup ketchup
- 1 tbsp. brown sugar
- 1 tbsp. mustard
- 1 tbsp. apple cider vinegar

Directions:
1.In a bowl, mix sugar with ketchup, mustard, stock, and vinegar and whisk well.
2.In your air fryer's pan, mix sausage slices with bell pepper, onion, and sweet and sour mix; toss and cook at 350 °F for 10 minutes. Divide into bowls and serve for lunch.
Nutrition:
Calories: 162;
Fat: 6;
Fiber: 9;
Carbs: 12;
Protein: 6

97.Fried Thai Salad

Preparation Time: 10 minutes
Cooking Time: 15 Minutes
Servings: 4

Ingredients:

- big shrimp; cooked, peeled and deveined
- 1 cup carrots; grated
- 1 cup red cabbage; shredded
- A handful cilantro; chopped.
- 1 small cucumber; chopped.
- Juice from 1 lime
- 1 tsp. red curry paste
- A pinch of salt and black pepper

Directions:

1.In a pan, mix cabbage with carrots, cucumber, and shrimp; toss, introduce in your air fryer and cook at 360 °F for 5 minutes.

2.Add salt, pepper, cilantro, lime juice, and red curry paste; toss again, divide among plates, and serve right away.

Nutrition:

Calories: 172;
Fat: 5;
Fiber: 7;
Carbs: 8;
Protein: 5

98.Seafood Stew

Preparation Time: 10 minutes
Cooking Time: 30 Minutes
Servings: 4
Ingredients:

- oz. white rice
- oz. sea bass fillet; skinless, boneless and chopped.
- oz. peas
- 1 red bell pepper; chopped.
- oz. white wine
- oz. water
- oz. squid pieces
- oz. mussels
- scallops
- oz. clams
- shrimp
- crayfish
- 1 tbsp. olive oil
- Salt and black pepper to the taste

Directions:

1.In your air fryer's pan, mix sea bass with shrimp, mussels, scallops, crayfish, clams, and squid.

2.Add the oil, salt, and pepper and toss to coat.

3.In a bowl, mix peas, salt, pepper, bell pepper, and rice and stir.

4.Add this over seafood, also add wine and water, place the pan in your air fryer and cook at 400 °F for 20 minutes, stirring halfway. Divide into bowls and serve for lunch.

Nutrition:

Calories: 300;
Fat: 12;
Fiber: 2;
Carbs: 23;
Protein: 25

99.Bacon Garlic Pizzas

Preparation Time: 10 minutes
Cooking Time: 20 Minutes
Servings: 4
Ingredients:

- dinner rolls; frozen
- bacon slices; cooked and chopped.
- 1 ¼ cups cheddar cheese; grated
- garlic cloves minced
- 1/2 tsp. oregano dried
- 1/2 tsp. garlic powder
- 1 cup tomato sauce
- Cooking spray

Directions:

1.Place dinner rolls on a working surface and press them to obtain 4 ovals.

2.Spray each oval with cooking spray; transfer them to your air fryer and cook them at 370 °F for 2 minutes.

3.Spread tomato sauce on each oval, divide garlic, sprinkle oregano, and garlic powder, and top with bacon and cheese.

4.Return pizzas to your heated air fryer and cook them at 370 °F for 8 minutes more. Serve them warm for lunch.

Nutrition:

Calories: 217;
Fat: 5;
Fiber: 8;
Carbs: 12;
Protein: 4

100.Chicken, Quinoa, Corn, Beans and Casserole

Preparation Time: 10 minutes

Cooking Time: 40 Minutes
Servings: 8
Ingredients:

- 1 cup quinoa; already cooked
- 2 cups chicken breast; cooked and shredded
- 1 tsp. chili powder
- 1 tsp. cumin; ground
- 2 cups mozzarella cheese; shredded
- oz. canned black beans
- oz. corn
- 1/2 cup cilantro; chopped.
- kale leaves; chopped.
- 1/2 cup green onions; chopped.
- 1 cup clean tomato sauce
- 1 cup clean salsa
- 1 tbsp. garlic powder
- Cooking spray
- jalapeno peppers; chopped.

Directions:

1.Spray a baking dish that fits your air fryer with cooking spray, add quinoa, chicken, black beans, corn, cilantro, kale, green onions, tomato sauce, salsa, chili powder, cumin, garlic powder, jalapenos, and mozzarella; toss,

2.introduce in your fryer and cook at 350 °F for 17 minutes.

3. Slice and serve warm for lunch.

Nutrition:

Calories: 365;
Fat: 12;
Fiber: 6;
Carbs: 22;
Protein: 26

101.Meatballs, Tomato Sauce

Preparation Time: 30 minutes
Cooking Time: 45 Minutes
Servings: 4
Ingredients:

- 1 lb. lean beef; ground
- green onions; chopped.
- garlic cloves; minced
- 1 egg yolk
- 1/4 cup bread crumbs
- 1 tbsp. olive oil
- oz. tomato sauce
- 1 tbsp. mustard
- Salt and black pepper to the taste

Directions:

1.In a bowl, mix beef with onion, garlic, egg yolk, bread crumbs, salt, and pepper, stir well, and shape medium meatballs out of this mix.

2.Grease meatballs with the oil, place them in your air fryer, and cook them at 400 °F for 10 minutes.

3.In a bowl, mix tomato sauce with mustard, whisk, add over meatballs, toss them and cook at 400 °F, for 5 minutes more. Divide meatballs and sauce between plates and serve for lunch.

Nutrition:

Calories: 300;
Fat: 8;
Fiber: 9;
Carbs: 16;
Protein: 5

Chapter 12.Sides

102.Pumpkin Ham Fritters

Preparation Time: 10 minutes
Cooking Time: 20 Minutes
Servings: 4
Ingredients

- 1 oz ham, chopped
- 1 cup dry pancake mix
- 1 egg
- 1 tbsp canned puree pumpkin
- 1 oz cheddar, shredded
- ½ tsp chili powder
- 1 tbsp of flour
- 1 oz beer
- 1 tbsp scallions, chopped

Directions

1.Preheat the Air fryer to 370 F and in a bowl, mix the pancake mix and chili powder. Add the egg, puree pumpkin, beer, shredded cheddar, ham, and scallions. Roll the mixture in 3 tbsp. of flour.
2.Arrange the balls into the basket and cook for 8 minutes. Drain on a paper towel before serving.

Nutrition:
Calories: 202;
Fat: 6;
Fiber: 3;
Carbs: 17;
Protein: 10

103.Spicy Hot Crab Cakes

Preparation Time: 20 minutes
Cooking Time: 20 Minutes
Servings: 6
Ingredients

- 1 lb. crab meat, shredded
- 4 eggs, beaten
- ½ cup breadcrumbs
- ⅓ cup finely chopped green onion
- ¼ cup parsley, chopped
- 1 tbsp mayonnaise
- 1 tsp sweet chili sauce
- ½ tsp paprika
- Salt and black pepper
- Olive oil to spray

Directions

1.In a bowl, add meat, eggs, crumbs, green onion, parsley, mayo, chili sauce, paprika, salt, and black pepper; mix well with hands.
2.Shape into 6 cakes and grease them lightly with oil. Arrange them in the fryer without overcrowding. Cook for 8 minutes at 400 F, turning once halfway through.

Nutrition:
Calories: 202;
Fat: 6;
Fiber: 3;
Carbs: 17;
Protein: 10

104.Pumpkin Wedges

Preparation Time: 30 minutes
Cooking Time: 50 Minutes
Servings: 3
Ingredients

- ½ pumpkin, washed and cut into wedges
- 1 tbsp paprika
- 1 whole lime, squeezed
- 1 cup paleo dressing
- 1 tbsp balsamic vinegar
- Salt and pepper to taste
- 1 tsp turmeric

Directions

1.Preheat your Air Fryer to 360 F. Add the pumpkin wedges to your air fryer's cooking basket, and cook for 20 minutes.
2.In a mixing bowl, mix lime juice, vinegar, turmeric, salt, pepper, and paprika to form a marinade.
3.Pour the marinade over the pumpkin, and cook for 5 more minutes.

Nutrition:
Calories: 202;
Fat: 6;
Fiber: 3;
Carbs: 17;
Protein: 10

105.Potato Chips Creamy Dip

Preparation Time: 25 minutes
Cooking Time: 70 Minutes
Servings: 3
Ingredients

- large potatoes

- 1 cup sour cream
- scallions, white part minced
- 1 tbsp olive oil.
- ½ tsp lemon juice
- salt and black pepper

Directions

1.Preheat the Air fryer to 350 F and slice the potatoes into thin slices; do not peel them. Soak them in water for 10 minutes, then dry them and spray with oil.

2.Fry the potato slices in two separate batches for 15 minutes; season with salt and pepper.

3.To prepare the dip, mix the sour cream, olive oil, the scallions, lemon juice, salt, and pepper.

Nutrition:

Calories: 202;
Fat: 6;
Fiber: 3;
Carbs: 17;
Protein: 10

106.Vegan Bok Choy Chips

Preparation Time: 10 minutes
Cooking Time: 20 Minutes
Servings: 2
Ingredients

- 1 tbsp olive oil
- 2 cups packed bok choy
- 1 tsp vegan seasoning
- 1 tbsp yeast flakes
- sea salt, to taste

Directions

1.In a bowl, mix oil, bok choy, yeast, and vegan seasoning. Dump the coated kale in the Air fryer's basket.

2.Set the temperature to 360 F and cook for 5 minutes. Shake after 3 minutes.

3.Serve sprinkled with sea salt.

Nutrition:

Calories: 202;
Fat: 6;
Fiber: 3;
Carbs: 17;
Protein: 10

107.Veggie & Ham Rolls with Walnuts

Preparation Time: 15 minutes
Cooking Time: 20 Minutes
Servings: 4
Ingredients

- rice leaves
- carrots
- slices ham
- oz walnuts, finely chopped
- 1 zucchini
- 1 clove garlic
- 1 tbsp olive oil
- 1 tbsp ginger powder
- ¼ cup basil leaves, finely chopped
- salt and pepper

Directions

1.In a cooking pan, pour olive oil and add the zucchini, carrots, garlic, ginger, and salt; cook on low heat for 10 minutes.

2.Add the basil and walnuts, and keep stirring. Soak the rice leaves in warm water. Then fold one side above the filling and roll in.

3.Cook the rolls in the preheated air fryer for 5 minutes at 300 F.

Nutrition:

Calories: 202;
Fat: 6;
Fiber: 3;
Carbs: 17;
Protein: 10

108.Rosemary Potato Chips

Preparation Time: 50 minutes
Cooking Time: 50 Minutes
Servings: 3
Ingredients

- whole potatoes, cut into thin slices
- ¼ cup olive oil
- 1 tbsp garlic
- ½ cup cream
- 1 tbsp rosemary

Directions

1.Preheat your Air Fryer to 390 F. In a bowl, add oil, garlic, and salt to form a marinade. In a separate bowl, add potato slices and top with cold water. Allow sitting for 30 minutes. Drain the slices and transfer them to the marinade.

2.Allow sitting for 30 minutes. Lay the potato slices onto your Air Fryer's cooking basket and cook for 20 minutes.

3.After 10 minutes, give the chips a turn, sprinkle with rosemary and serve.

Nutrition:

Calories: 202;
Fat: 6;
Fiber: 3;
Carbs: 17;
Protein: 10

109.Simple Cheese Sandwich

Preparation Time: 20 minutes
Cooking Time: 20 Minutes
Servings: 1
Ingredients

- 1 tbsp Parmesan, shredded
- scallions
- 1 tbsp butter
- 4 slices bread
- ¾ cup Cheddar cheese

Directions
1.Preheat your Air Fryer to 360 F. Lay the bread slices on a flat surface. On one slice, spread the exposed side with butter, followed by cheddar and scallions. On the other slice, spread butter and then sprinkle cheese.
2.Bring the buttered sides together to form sand. Place the sandwich in your Air Fryer's cooking basket and cook for 10 minutes. Serve with berry sauce.
Nutrition:
Calories: 202;
Fat: 6;
Fiber: 3;
Carbs: 17;
Protein: 10

110.Cheesy Cheddar Biscuits

Preparation Time: 35 minutes
Cooking Time: 50 minutes
Servings: 8
Ingredients

- ½ cup + 1 tbsp butter
- 1 tbsp sugar
- 2 cups flour
- 1 ⅓ cups buttermilk
- ½ cup Cheddar, grated

Directions
1.Preheat your Air Fryer to 380 F. Lay a parchment paper on a baking plate. In a bowl, mix sugar, flour, ½ cup butter, cheese, and buttermilk to form a batter. Make 8 balls from the batter and roll in flour.
2.Place the balls in your air fryer's cooking basket and flatten into biscuit shapes. Sprinkle cheese and the remaining butter on top. Cook for 30 minutes, tossing every 10 minutes. Serve warm.
Nutrition:
Calories: 202;
Fat: 6;
Fiber: 3;
Carbs: 17;
Protein: 10

111.Roasted Cashew Delight

Preparation Time: 20 minutes
Cooking Time: 40 Minutes
Servings: 12
Ingredients

- 2 cups cashews
- 1 tbsp liquid smoke
- 1 tsp salt
- 1 tbsp molasses

Directions
1.Preheat your Air Fryer to 360 F.
2.In a bowl, add salt, liquid, molasses, and cashews; toss to coat well.
3.Place the coated cashews in your Air Fryer's cooking basket and cook for 10 minutes, shaking the basket every 5 minutes.
Nutrition:
Calories: 202;
Fat: 6;
Fiber: 3;
Carbs: 17;
Protein: 10

112.Hearty Grilled Ham and Cheese

Preparation Time: 15 minutes
Cooking Time: 40 Minutes
Servings: 2
Ingredients

- slices bread
- ¼ cup butter
- slices ham
- slices cheese

Directions
1.Preheat your Air Fryer to 360 degrees F.
2. Place 2 bread slices on a flat surface.
3.Spread butter on the exposed surfaces.
4.Lay cheese and ham on two of the slices.
5. Cover with the other 2 slices to form sandwiches.
6. Place the sandwiches in the cooking basket and cook for 5 minutes.

Nutrition:
Calories: 202;
Fat: 6;
Fiber: 3;
Carbs: 17;
Protein: 10

113.Parsnip Fries

Preparation Time: 15 minutes
Cooking Time: 20 Minutes
Servings: 3
Ingredients

- large parsnips
- ¼ cup flour
- ¼ cup olive oil
- ¼ cup water
- A pinch of salt

Directions
1.Preheat the Air Fryer to 390 F and cut the parsnip to a half-inch by 3 inches. In a bowl, mix the flour, olive oil, water, and parsnip. Mix well and coat. Line the fries in the air fryer and cook for 15 minutes.
2.Serve with yogurt and garlic paste.
Nutrition:
Calories: 202;
Fat: 6;
Fiber: 3;
Carbs: 17;
Protein: 10

114.Tender Eggplant Fries

Preparation Time: 20 minutes
Cooking Time: 30 Minutes
Servings: 2
Ingredients

- 1 eggplant, sliced
- 1 tsp olive oil
- 1 tsp soy sauce
- Salt to taste

Directions
1.Preheat your Air Fryer to 400 F. Make a marinade of 1 tsp oil, soy sauce, and salt.
2.Mix well. Add in the eggplant slices and let stand for 5 minutes.
3.Place the prepared eggplant slices in your Air Fryer's cooking basket and cook for 5 minutes.
4.Serve with a drizzle of maple syrup.
Nutrition:
Calories: 202;
Fat: 6;
Fiber: 3;
Carbs: 17;
Protein: 10

115.Cabbage Canapes

Preparation Time: 15 minutes
Cooking Time: 30 minutes
Servings: 2
Ingredients

- 1 whole cabbage, washed and cut into rounds
- 1 cube Amul cheese
- ½ carrot, cubed
- ¼ onion, cubed
- ¼ capsicum, cubed
- Fresh basil to garnish

Directions
1.Preheat your Air Fryer to 360 F. Using a bowl, mix onion, carrot, capsicum, and cheese. Toss to coat everything evenly. Add cabbage rounds to the Air Fryer's cooking basket.
2.Top with the veggie mixture and cook for 5 minutes. Serve with a garnish of fresh basil.
Nutrition:
Calories: 202;
Fat: 6;
Fiber: 3;
Carbs: 17;
Protein: 10

116.Crispy Bacon with Butterbean Dip

Preparation Time: 10 minutes
Cooking Time: 20 Minutes
Servings: 2
Ingredients

- 1 -14 oz can butter beans
- 1 tbsp chives
- ½ oz feta
- Pepper to taste
- 1 tsp olive oil
- ½ oz bacon, sliced

Directions
1.Preheat your Air Fryer to 340 F. Blend beans, oil, and pepper using a blender.

2.Arrange bacon slices on your Air Fryer's cooking basket. Sprinkle chives on top and cook for 10 minutes.
3.Add feta cheese to the butter bean blend and stir.
4.Serve bacon with the dip.

Nutrition:
Calories: 202;
Fat: 6;
Fiber: 3;
Carbs: 17;
Protein: 10

117.Almond French Beans

Preparation Time: 25 minutes
Cooking Time: 35 minutes
Servings: 5
Ingredients

- 1 ½ pound French beans, washed and drained
- 1 tbsp salt
- 1 tbsp pepper
- ½ pound shallots, chopped
- tbsp olive oil
- ½ cup almonds, toasted

Directions
1.Preheat your Air Fryer to 400 F. Put a pan over medium heat,
2.Mix beans in hot water and boil until tender, about 5-6 minutes.
3.Mix the boiled beans with oil, shallots, salt, and pepper.
4.Add the mixture to your Air Fryer's cooking basket and cook for 20 minutes.
5.Serve with almonds and enjoy!

Nutrition:
Calories: 202;
Fat: 6;
Fiber: 3;
Carbs: 17;
Protein: 10

118.Spicy Cajun Shrimp

Preparation Time: 15 minutes
Cooking Time: 20 Minutes
Servings: 3
Ingredients

- ½ pound shrimp, sauce and deveined
- ½ tsp cajun seasoning
- Salt as needed
- 1 tbsp olive oil
- ¼ tsp pepper
- ¼ tsp paprika

Directions
1.Preheat your Air Fryer to 390 F.
2.Using a bowl, make the marinade by mixing paprika, salt, pepper, oil, and seasoning. Cut shrimp and cover with marinade.
3.Place the prepared shrimp in your Air Fryer's cooking basket and cook for 10 minutes, flipping halfway through.

Nutrition:
Calories: 202;
Fat: 6;
Fiber: 3;
Carbs: 17;
Protein: 10

119.Roasted Brussels Sprouts

Preparation Time: 25 minutes
Cooking Time: 20 Minutes
Servings: 4
Ingredients

- 1 block brussels sprouts
- ½ tsp garlic, chopped
- tbsp olive oil
- ½ tsp pepper
- Salt to taste

Directions
1.Wash the Brussels thoroughly under cold water and trim off the outer leaves, keeping only the head of the sprouts.
2.In a bowl, mix oil and garlic. Season with salt and pepper. Add prepared sprouts to this mixture and let rest for 5 minutes.
3.Place the coated sprouts in your air fryer's cooking basket and cook for 15 minutes.

Nutrition:
Calories: 202;
Fat: 6;
Fiber: 3;
Carbs: 17;
Protein: 10

Chapter 13.Poultry

120.Deviled Chicken

Preparation Time: 10 minutes
Cooking Time: 40 minutes
Servings: 8
Ingredients

- 2 tablespoons butter
- cloves garlic, chopped
- 1 cup dijon mustard
- 1/2 teaspoon cayenne pepper
- 1 1/2 cups panko breadcrumbs
- 3/4 cup parmesan, freshly grated
- 1/4 cup chives, chopped
- 2 teaspoons paprika
- small bone-in chicken thighs, skin removed

Directions:

1.Toss the chicken thighs with crumbs, cheese, chives, butter, and spices in a bowl and mix well to coat.
2.Transfer the chicken along with its spice mix to a baking pan.
3.Press the "power button" of the air fry oven and turn the dial to select the "air fry" mode.
4.Press the time button and again turn the dial to set the cooking time to 40 minutes.
5.Now push the temp button and rotate the dial to set the temperature at 350 degrees f.
6.Once preheated, place the baking pan inside and close its lid.
7.Serve warm.

Nutrition:

Calories 380
Total fat 20 g
Saturated fat 5 g
Cholesterol 151 mg
Sodium 686 mg
Total carbs 33 g
Fiber 1 g
Sugar 1.2 g
Protein 21 g

121.Marinated Chicken Parmesan

Preparation Time: 10 minutes
Cooking Time: 20 minutes
Servings: 4
Ingredients

- 2 cups breadcrumbs
- 1 teaspoon dried oregano
- 1/2 teaspoon garlic powder
- 2 teaspoons paprika
- 1/2 teaspoon salt
- 1/2 teaspoon black pepper
- 4 egg whites
- 1/2 cup skim milk
- 1/2 cup flour
- oz. Chicken breast halves
- Cooking spray
- 1 jar marinara sauce
- 3/4 cup mozzarella cheese, shredded
- 2 tablespoons parmesan, shredded

Directions:

1.Whisk the flour with all the spices in a bowl and beat the eggs in another.
2.Coat the pounded chicken with flour, then dip in the egg whites.
3.Dredge the chicken breast through the crumbs well.
4.Spread marinara sauce in a baking dish and place the crusted chicken on it.
5.Drizzle cheese on top of the chicken.
6.Press the "power button" of the air fry oven and turn the dial to select the "bake" mode.
7.Press the time button and again turn the dial to set the cooking time to 20 minutes.
8.Now push the temp button and rotate the dial to set the temperature at 400 degrees f.
9.Once preheated, place the baking pan inside and close its lid.
10. Serve warm.

Nutrition:

Calories 361
Total fat 16.3 g
Saturated fat 4.9 g
Cholesterol 114 mg
Sodium 515 mg
Total carbs 19.3 g
Fiber 0.1 g
Sugar 18.2 g
Protein 33.3 g

122.Rosemary Lemon Chicken

Preparation Time: 10 minutes

Cooking Time: 45 minutes
Servings: 8
Ingredients
- 4-lb. (1814.37g) Chicken, cut into pieces
- Salt and black pepper, to taste
- Flour for dredging
- 2 tablespoons olive oil
- 1 large onion, sliced
- Peel of ½ lemon
- large garlic cloves, minced
- 1 1/2 teaspoons rosemary leaves
- 1 tablespoon honey
- 1/4 cup lemon juice
- 1 cup chicken broth

Directions:
1.Dredges the chicken through the flour, then place in the baking pan.
2.Whisk broth with the rest of the ingredients in a bowl.
3.Pour this mixture over the dredged chicken in the pan.
4.Press the "power button" of the air fry oven and turn the dial to select the "bake" mode.
5.Press the time button and again turn the dial to set the cooking time to 45 minutes.
6.Now push the temp button and rotate the dial to set the temperature at 400 degrees f.
7.Once preheated, place the baking pan inside and close its lid.
8.Baste the chicken with its sauce every 15 minutes.
9.Serve warm.
Nutrition:
Calories 405
Total fat 22.7 g
Saturated fat 6.1 g
Cholesterol 4 mg
Sodium 227 mg
Total carbs 26.1 g
Fiber 1.4 g
Sugar 0.9 g
Protein 45.2 g

123.Garlic Chicken Potatoes

Preparation Time: 10 minutes
Cooking Time: 30 minutes
Servings: 4
Ingredients
- lbs. (907.185g) Red potatoes, quartered
- 1 tablespoons olive oil
- 1/2 teaspoon cumin seeds
- Salt and black pepper, to taste
- garlic cloves, chopped
- 2 tablespoons brown sugar
- 1 lemon (1/2 juiced and 1/2 cut into wedges)
- Pinch of red pepper flakes
- skinless, boneless chicken breasts
- 2 tablespoons cilantro, chopped

Directions:
1.Place the chicken, lemon, garlic, and potatoes in a baking pan.
2.Toss the spices, herbs, oil, and sugar in a bowl.
3.Add this mixture to the chicken and veggies, then toss well to coat.
4.Press the "power button" of the air fry oven and turn the dial to select the "bake" mode.
5.Press the time button and again turn the dial to set the cooking time to 30 minutes.
6.Now push the temp button and rotate the dial to set the temperature at 400 degrees f.
7.Once preheated, place the baking pan inside and close its lid.
8.Serve warm.
Nutrition:
Calories 545
Total fat 36.4 g
Saturated fat 10.1 g
Cholesterol 200 mg
Sodium 272 mg
Total carbs 40.7 g
Fiber 0.2 g
Sugar 0.1 g
Protein 42.5 g

124.Chicken Potato Bake

Preparation Time: 10 minutes
Cooking Time: 25 minutes
Servings: 4
Ingredients
- potatoes, diced
- 1 tablespoon garlic, minced
- 1.5 tablespoons olive oil
- 1/8 teaspoon salt
- 1/8 teaspoon pepper

- 1.5 lbs. (680.389g) Boneless skinless chicken
- 3/4 cup mozzarella cheese, shredded
- Parsley chopped

Directions:

1.Toss chicken and potatoes with all the spices and oil in a baking pan.
2.Drizzle the cheese on top of the chicken and potato.
3.Press the "power button" of the air fry oven and turn the dial to select the "bake" mode.
4.Press the time button and again turn the dial to set the cooking time to 25 minutes.
5.Now push the temp button and rotate the dial to set the temperature at 375 degrees f.
6.Once preheated, place the baking pan inside and close its lid.
7.Serve warm.

Nutrition:

Calories 695
Total fat 17.5 g
Saturated fat 4.8 g
Cholesterol 283 mg
Sodium 355 mg
Total carbs 26.4 g
Fiber 1.8 g
Sugar 0.8 g
Protein 117.4 g

125.Spanish Chicken Bake

Preparation Time: 10 minutes
Cooking Time: 25 minutes
Servings: 4
Ingredients

- ½ onion, quartered
- ½ red onion, quartered
- ½ lb. (226.8g) Potatoes, quartered
- garlic cloves
- tomatoes, quartered
- 1/8 cup chorizo
- ¼ teaspoon paprika powder
- chicken thighs, boneless
- ¼ teaspoon dried oregano
- ½ green bell pepper, julienned
- Salt
- Black pepper

Directions:

1.Toss chicken, veggies, and all the ingredients in a baking tray.
2.Press the "power button" of the air fry oven and turn the dial to select the "bake" mode.
3.Press the time button and again turn the dial to set the cooking time to 25 minutes.
4.Now push the temp button and rotate the dial to set the temperature at 425 degrees f.
5.Once preheated, place the baking pan inside and close its lid.
6.Serve warm.

Nutrition:

Calories 301
Total fat 8.9 g
Saturated fat 4.5 g
Cholesterol 57 mg
Sodium 340 mg
Total carbs 24.7 g
Fiber 1.2 g
Sugar 1.3 g
Protein 15.3 g

126.Chicken Pasta Bake

Preparation Time: 10 minutes
Cooking Time: 22 minutes
Servings: 4
Ingredients

- 9oz penne, boiled
- 1 onion, roughly chopped
- chicken breasts, cut into strips
- 1 tablespoon olive oil
- 1 tablespoon paprika
- Salt and black pepper

Sauce

- 1¾oz butter
- 1¾oz plain flour
- 1 pint 6 fl oz hot milk
- 1 teaspoon dijon mustard
- 3½oz parmesan cheese, grated
- large tomatoes, deseeded and cubed

Directions:

1.Butter a casserole dish and toss chicken with pasta, onion, oil, paprika, salt, and black pepper in it.
2.Prepare the sauce in a suitable pan. Add butter and melt over moderate heat.
3.Stir in flour and whisk well for 2 minutes, then pour in hot milk.
4.Mix until smooth, then add tomatoes, mustard, and cheese.

5.Toss well and pour this sauce over the chicken mix in the casserole dish.
6.Press the "power button" of the air fry oven and turn the dial to select the "bake" mode.
7.Press the time button and again turn the dial to set the cooking time to 20 minutes.
8.Now push the temp button and rotate the dial to set the temperature at 375 degrees f.
9.Once preheated, place the casserole dish inside and close its lid.
10. Serve warm.

Nutrition:

Calories 548
Total fat 22.9 g
Saturated fat 9 g
Cholesterol 105 mg
Sodium 350 mg
Total carbs 17.5 g
Sugar 10.9 g
Fiber 6.3 g
Protein 40.1 g

127.Creamy Chicken Casserole

Preparation Time: 10 minutes
Cooking Time: 45 minutes
Servings: 6
Ingredients

- Chicken and mushroom casserole:
- 1/2 lbs. (1133.98g) Chicken breasts, cut into strips
- 1 1/2 teaspoon salt
- 1/4 teaspoon black pepper
- 1 cup all-purpose flour
- 1 tablespoon olive oil
- 1-lb. (453.592g) White mushrooms, sliced
- 1 medium onion, diced
- garlic cloves, minced

Sauce:

- tablespoon unsalted butter
- tablespoon all-purpose flour
- 1 1/2 cups chicken broth
- 1 tablespoon lemon juice
- 1 cup half and half cream

Directions:

1.Butter a casserole dish and toss in chicken with mushrooms and all the casserole ingredients.
2.Prepare the sauce in a suitable pan. Add butter and melt over moderate heat.
3.Stir in flour and whisk well for 2 minutes, then pour in milk, lemon juice, and cream.
4.Mix well and pour milk this sauce over the chicken mix in the casserole dish.
5.Press the "power button" of the air fry oven and turn the dial to select the "bake" mode.
6.Press the time button and again turn the dial to set the cooking time to 45 minutes.
7.Now push the temp button and rotate the dial to set the temperature at 350 degrees f.
8.Once preheated, place the casserole dish inside and close its lid.
9.Serve warm.

Nutrition:

Calories 409
Total fat 50.5 g
Saturated fat 11.7 g
Cholesterol 58 mg
Sodium 463 mg
Total carbs 9.9 g
Fiber 1.5 g
Sugar 0.3 g
Protein 29.3 g

128.Italian Chicken Bake

Preparation Time: 10 minutes
Cooking Time: 25 minutes
Servings: 6
Ingredients:

- ¾ lbs. (340.194g) Chicken breasts
- 2 tablespoons pesto sauce
- ½ (14 oz) can tomatoes, diced
- 1 cup mozzarella cheese, shredded
- 2 tablespoon fresh basil, chopped

Directions:

1.Place the flattened chicken breasts in a baking pan and top them with pesto.
2.Add tomatoes, cheese, and basil on top of each chicken piece.
3.Press the "power button" of the air fry oven and turn the dial to select the "bake" mode.
4.Press the time button and again turn the dial to set the cooking time to 25 minutes.
5.Now push the button and rotate the dial to set the temperature at 355 degrees f.
6.Once preheated, place the baking dish inside and close its lid.

7.Serve warm.

Nutrition:

Calories 537
Total fat 19.8 g
Saturated fat 1.4 g
Cholesterol 10 mg
Sodium 719 mg
Total carbs 25.1 g
Fiber 0.9 g
Sugar 1.4 g
Protein 37.8 g

129.Pesto Chicken Bake

Preparation Time: 10 minutes
Cooking Time: 35 minutes
Servings: 3

Ingredients

- chicken breasts
- 1 (6 oz.) Jar basil pesto
- medium fresh tomatoes, sliced
- mozzarella cheese slices

Directions:

1.Spread the tomato slices in a casserole dish and top them with chicken.
2.Add pesto and cheese on top of the chicken and spread evenly.
3.Press the "power button" of the air fry oven and turn the dial to select the "air fry" mode.
4.Press the time button and again turn the dial to set the cooking time to 30 minutes.
5.Now push the temp button and rotate the dial to set the temperature at 350 degrees f.
6.Once preheated, place the casserole dish inside and close its lid.
7.After it is baked, switch the oven to broil mode and broil for 5 minutes.
8.Serve warm.

Nutrition:

Calories 452
Total fat 4 g
Saturated fat 2 g
Cholesterol 65 mg
Sodium 220 mg
Total carbs 23.1 g
Fiber 0.3 g
Sugar 1 g
Protein 26g

Chapter 14.Poultry 2

130.Baked Duck

Preparation Time: 10 minutes
Cooking Time: 20 minutes
Servings: 6
Ingredients

- 1 ½ sprig of fresh rosemary
- ½ nutmeg
- Black pepper
- Juice from 1 orange
- 1 whole duck
- cloves garlic, chopped
- 1 ½ red onions, chopped
- A few stalks celery
- 1 ½ carrot
- piece fresh ginger
- 1 ½ bay leaves
- lbs. (907.185g) Piper potatoes
- 2 cups chicken stock

Directions:

1.Place duck in a large cooking pot and add broth along with all the ingredients.
2.Cook this duck for 2 hours on a simmer, then transfer to the baking tray.
3.Press the "power button" of the air fry oven and turn the dial to select the "air fry" mode.
4.Press the time button and again turn the dial to set the cooking time to 20 minutes.
5.Now push the temp button and rotate the dial to set the temperature at 350 degrees f.
6.Once preheated, place the baking tray inside and close its lid.
7.Serve warm.

Nutrition:

Calories 308
Total fat 20.5 g
Saturated fat 3 g
Cholesterol 42 mg
Sodium 688 mg
Total carbs 40.3 g
Sugar 1.4 g
Fiber 4.3 g
Protein 49 g

131.Roasted Goose

Preparation Time: 10 minutes
Cooking Time: 40 minutes
Servings: 12
Ingredients

- lbs. (3628.74g) Goose
- Juice of a lemon
- Salt and pepper
- 1/2 yellow onion, peeled and chopped
- 1 head garlic, peeled and chopped
- 1/2 cup wine
- 1 teaspoon dried thyme

Directions:

1.Place the goose in a baking tray and whisk the rest of the ingredients in a bowl.
2.Pour this thick sauce over the goose and brush it liberally.
3.Press the "power button" of the air fry oven and turn the dial to select the "air roast" mode.
4.Press the time button and again turn the dial to set the cooking time to 40 minutes.
5.Now push the temp button and rotate to set the temperature at 355 degrees f.
6.Once preheated, place the casserole dish inside and close its lid.
7.Serve warm.

Nutrition:

Calories 231
Total fat 20.1 g
Saturated fat 2.4 g
Cholesterol 110 mg
Sodium 941 mg
Total carbs 20.1 g
Fiber 0.9 g
Sugar 1.4 g
Protein 14.6 g

132.Christmas Roast Goose

Preparation Time: 10 minutes
Cooking Time: 60 minutes
Servings: 12
Ingredients

- goose
- lemons, sliced
- 1 ½ lime, sliced
- ½ teaspoon Chinese five-spice powder
- ½ handful parsley, chopped

- ½ handful sprigs, chopped
- ½ handful thyme, chopped
- ½ handful sage, chopped
- 1 ½ tablespoon clear honey
- ½ tablespoon thyme leaves

Directions:

1.Place the goose in a baking dish and brush it with honey.
2.Set the lemon and lime slices on top of the goose.
3.Add all the herbs and spice powder over the lemon slices.
4.Press the "power button" of the air fry oven and turn the dial to select the "air roast" mode.
5.Press the time button and again turn the dial to set the cooking time to 60 minutes.
6.Now push the temp button and rotate the dial to set the temperature at 375 degrees f.
7.Once preheated, place the baking dish inside and close its lid.
8.Serve warm.

Nutrition:

Calories 472
Total fat 11.1 g
Saturated fat 5.8 g
Cholesterol 610 mg
Sodium 749 mg
Total carbs 19.9 g
Fiber 0.2 g
Sugar 0.2 g
Protein 13.5 g

133.Chicken Kebabs

Preparation Time: 10 minutes
Cooking Time: 20 minutes
Servings: 2
Ingredients

- oz skinless chicken breasts, cubed
- 2 tablespoons soy sauce
- ½ zucchini sliced
- 1 tablespoon chicken seasoning
- 1 teaspoon bbq seasoning
- Salt and pepper to taste
- ½ green pepper sliced
- ½ red pepper sliced
- ½ yellow pepper sliced
- ¼ red onion sliced
- cherry tomatoes
- Cooking spray

Directions:

1.Toss chicken and veggies with all the spices and seasoning in a bowl.
2.Alternatively, thread them on skewers and place these skewers in the air fryer basket.
3.Press the "power button" of the air fry oven and turn the dial to select the "air fry" mode.
4.Press the time button and again turn the dial to set the cooking time to 20 minutes.
5.Now push the temp button and rotate the dial to set the temperature at 350 degrees f.
6.Once preheated, place the baking dish inside and close its lid.
7.Flip the skewers when cooked halfway through, then resume cooking.
8.Serve warm.

Nutrition:

Calories 327
Total fat 3.5 g
Saturated fat 0.5 g
Cholesterol 162 mg
Sodium 142 mg
Total carbs 33.6 g
Fiber 0.4 g
Sugar 0.5 g
Protein 24.5 g

134.Asian Chicken Kebabs

Preparation Time: 10 minutes
Cooking Time: 12 minutes
Servings: 6
Ingredients

- lbs (907.185g) Chicken breasts, cubed
- 1/2 cup soy sauce
- cloves garlic, crushed
- 1 teaspoon fresh ginger, grated
- 1/2 cup golden sweetener
- 1 red pepper, chopped
- 1/2 red onion, chopped
- mushrooms, halved
- 2 cups zucchini, chopped

Directions:

1.Toss chicken and veggies with all the spices and seasoning in a bowl.
2.Alternatively, thread them on skewers and place these skewers in the air fryer basket.

3.Press the "power button" of the air fry oven and turn the dial to select the "air fry" mode.
4.Press the time button and again turn the dial to set the cooking time to 12 minutes.
5.Now push the temp button and rotate the dial to set the temperature at 380 degrees f.
6.Once preheated, place the baking dish inside and close its lid.
7.Flip the skewers when cooked halfway through, then resume cooking.
8.Serve warm.

Nutrition:

Calories 353
Total fat 7.5 g
Saturated fat 1.1 g
Cholesterol 20 mg
Sodium 297 mg
Total carbs 10.4 g
Fiber 0.2 g
Sugar 0.1 g
Protein 13.1 g

135.Kebab Tavuk Sheesh

Preparation Time: 10 minutes
Cooking Time: 10 minutes
Servings: 2
Ingredients

- 1/4 cup plain yogurt
- 1 tablespoon garlic, minced
- 1 tablespoon tomato paste
- 1 tablespoon olive oil
- 1 tablespoon lemon juice
- 1 teaspoon salt
- 1 teaspoon ground cumin
- 1 teaspoon smoked paprika
- 1/2 teaspoon ground cinnamon
- 1/2 teaspoon ground black pepper
- 1/2 teaspoon cayenne
- 1 lb. (453.592g) Boneless skinless chicken thighs, quartered

Directions:

1.Mix chicken with yogurt and all the seasonings in a bowl.
2.Marinate the yogurt chicken for 30 minutes in the refrigerator.
3.Thread chicken pieces on the skewers and place these skewers in the air fryer basket.
4.Press the "power button" of the air fry oven and turn the dial to select the "air fry" mode.
5.Press the time button and again turn the dial to set the cooking time to 10 minutes.
6.Now push the temp button and rotate the dial to set the temperature at 370 degrees f.
7.Once preheated, place the baking dish inside and close its lid.
8.Flip the skewers when cooked halfway through, then resume cooking.
9.Serve warm.

Nutrition:

Calories 248
Total fat 13 g
Saturated fat 7 g
Cholesterol 387 mg
Sodium 353 mg
Total carbs 1 g
Fiber 0.4 g
Sugar 1 g
Protein 29 g

136.Chicken Mushroom Kebab

Preparation Time: 10 minutes
Cooking Time: 15 minutes
Servings: 4
Ingredients

- 1/3 cup honey
- 1/3 cup soy sauce
- Salt, to taste
- mushrooms chop in half
- bell peppers, cubed
- chicken breasts diced

Directions:

1.Toss chicken, mushrooms, and veggies with all the honey and seasoning in a bowl.
2.Alternatively, thread them on skewers and place these skewers in the air fryer basket.
3.Press the "power button" of the air fry oven and turn the dial to select the "air fry" mode.
4.Press the time button and again turn the dial to set the cooking time to 15 minutes.
5.Now push the temp button and rotate the dial to set the temperature at 350 degrees f.
6.Once preheated, place the baking dish inside and close its lid.
7.Flip the skewers when cooked halfway through, then resume cooking.
8.Serve warm.

Nutrition:

Calories 457
Total fat 19.1 g

Saturated fat 11 g
Cholesterol 262 mg
Sodium 557 mg
Total carbs 18.9 g
Sugar 1.2 g
Fiber 1.7 g
Protein 32.5 g

137.Chicken Fajita Skewers

Preparation Time: 10 minutes
Cooking Time: 8 minutes
Servings: 2
Ingredients

- 1 lb. (453.592g) Chicken breasts, diced
- 1 tablespoon lemon juice
- 1 teaspoon chili powder
- 1 teaspoon cumin
- 1 orange bell pepper, cut into squares
- 1 red bell pepper, cut into squares
- 1 tablespoon olive oil
- 1 teaspoon garlic powder
- 1 large red onion, cut into squares
- 1 teaspoon salt
- 1 teaspoon ground black pepper
- 1 teaspoon oregano
- 1 teaspoon parsley flakes
- 1 teaspoon paprika

Directions:
1.Toss chicken and veggies with all the spices and seasoning in a bowl.
2.Alternatively, thread them on skewers and place these skewers in the air fryer basket.
3.Press the "power button" of the air fry oven and turn the dial to select the "air fry" mode.
4.Press the time button and again turn the dial to set the cooking time to 8 minutes.
5.Now push the temp button and rotate the dial to set the temperature at 360 degrees f.
6.Once preheated, place the baking dish inside and close its lid.
7.Flip the skewers when cooked halfway through, then resume cooking.
8.Serve warm.
Nutrition:
Calories 392
Total fat 16.1 g
Saturated fat 2.3 g
Cholesterol 231 mg
Sodium 466 mg
Total carbs 13.9 g
Sugar 0.6 g
Fiber 0.9 g
Protein 48 g

138.Zucchini Chicken Kebabs

Preparation Time: 10 minutes
Cooking Time: 16 minutes
Servings: 4
Ingredients

- 1 large zucchini, cut into squares
- chicken breasts boneless, skinless, cubed
- 1 onion yellow, cut into squares
- 1.5 cup grape tomatoes
- 1 clove garlic minced
- 1 lemon juiced
- 1/4 c olive oil
- 1 tablespoon olive oil
- 1 tablespoon red wine vinegar
- 1 teaspoon oregano

Directions:
1.Toss chicken and veggies with all the spices and seasoning in a bowl.
2.Alternatively, thread them on skewers and place these skewers in the air fryer basket.
3.Press the "power button" of the air fry oven and turn the dial to select the "air fry" mode.
4.Press the time button and again turn the dial to set the cooking time to 16 minutes.
5.Now push the temp button and rotate the dial to set the temperature at 380 degrees f.
6.Once preheated, place the baking dish inside and close its lid.
7.Flip the skewers when cooked halfway through, then resume cooking.
8.Serve warm.
Nutrition:
Calories 321
Total fat 7.4 g
Saturated fat 4.6 g
Cholesterol 105 mg
Sodium 353 mg
Total carbs 19.4 g
Sugar 6.5 g
Fiber 2.7 g
Protein 37.2 g

139.Chicken Soy Skewers

Preparation Time: 10 minutes
Cooking Time: 7 minutes
Servings: 4
Ingredients

- 1-lb. (453.592g) Boneless chicken tenders, diced
- 1/2 cup soy sauce
- 1/2 cup pineapple juice
- 1/4 cup sesame seed oil
- garlic cloves, chopped
- scallions, chopped
- 1 tablespoon grated ginger
- 2 teaspoons toasted sesame seeds
- Black pepper

Directions:

1.Toss chicken with all the sauces and seasonings in a baking pan.
2.Press the "power button" of the air fry oven and turn the dial to select the "air fry" mode.
3.Press the time button and again turn the dial to set the cooking time to 7 minutes.
4.Now push the temp button and rotate the dial to set the temperature at 390 degrees f.
5.Once preheated, place the baking dish inside and close its lid.
6.Serve warm.

Nutrition:

Calories 248
Total fat 15.7 g
Saturated fat 2.7 g
Cholesterol 75 mg
Sodium 94 mg
Total carbs 31.4 g
Fiber 0.4 g
Sugar 3.1 g
Protein 24.9 g

Chapter 15.Vegetables

140.Mushroom and Feta Frittata

Preparation Time: 5 minutes
Cooking Time: 30 minutes
Servings: 4
Ingredients:

- 2 cups button mushrooms
- red onion
- 2 tablespoons olive oil
- 2 tablespoons feta cheese, crumbled
- Pinch of salt
- 2 eggs
- Cooking spray

Directions:
1.Add olive oil to a pan and sauté mushrooms over medium heat until tender. Remove from heat and pan so that they can cool. Preheat your air fryer to 330°F.
2.Add cracked eggs into a bowl, and whisk them, adding a pinch of salt. Coat an 8-inch heat resistant baking dish with cooking spray. Add the eggs into the baking dish, then onion and mushroom mixture, and then add feta cheese.
3.Place the baking dish into the air fryer for 30-minutes and serve warm.
Nutrition:
Calories: 246 kcal/Cal
Total Fat: 12.3 g
Carbohydrates: 9.2 g
Protein: 10.3 g

141.Cauliflower Pizza Crust

Preparation Time: 26 minutes
Cooking Time: 20 minutes
Servings: 2
Ingredients:

- 1 (12-oz.) Steamer bag cauliflower
- 1 large egg.
- ½ cup shredded sharp cheddar cheese.
- tbsp. Blanched finely ground almond flour
- 1 tsp. Italian blend seasoning

Directions:
1.Cook cauliflower according to package instructions. Remove from bag and place into cheesecloth or paper towel to remove excess water. Place cauliflower into a large bowl.
2.Cut a piece of parchment to fit your air fryer basket. Press cauliflower into a 6-inch round circle. Place into the air fryer basket. Adjust the temperature to 360°F and set the timer for 11 minutes. After 7 minutes, flip the pizza crust
3.Add preferred toppings to the pizza. Place back into the air fryer basket and cook for an additional 4 minutes or until fully cooked and golden. Serve right away.
Nutrition:
Calories: 230 kcal/Cal
Protein: 14.9 g
Fiber: 4.7 g
Fat: 14.2 g
Carbohydrates: 10.0 g

142.Olives and Artichokes

Preparation Time: 20 minutes
Cooking Time: 15 minutes
Servings: 4
Ingredients:

- oz. canned artichoke hearts, drained
- ½ cup tomato sauce
- 2 cups black olives, pitted
- garlic cloves; minced
- 1 tbsp. Olive oil
- 1 tsp. Garlic powder

Directions:
1.In a pan that fits your air fryer, mix the olives with the artichokes and the other ingredients, toss,
2.put the pan in the fryer and cook at 350°f for 15 minutes
3.Divide the mix between plates and serve.
Nutrition:
Calories: 180 kcal/Cal
Fat: 4 g
Fiber: 3 g
Carbohydrates: 5 g
Protein: 6 g

143.Lemon Asparagus

Preparation Time: 17 minutes
Cooking Time: 12 minutes
Servings: 4
Ingredients:

- 1 lb. Asparagus, trimmed
- garlic cloves; minced

- 1 tbsp. Parmesan, grated
- 1 tbsp. Olive oil
- Juice of 1 lemon
- A pinch of salt and black pepper

Directions:

1.Take a bowl and mix the asparagus with the rest of the ingredients and toss.

2.Put the asparagus in your air fryer's basket and cook at 390°F for 12 minutes. Divide between plates and serve!

Nutrition:

Calories: 175 kcal/Cal
Fat: 5 g
Fiber: 2 g
Carbohydrates: 4 g
Protein: 8 g

144.Savory Cabbage and Tomatoes

Preparation Time: 20 minutes
Cooking Time: 15 minutes
Servings: 4
Ingredients:

- spring onions; chopped.
- 1 savoy cabbage, shredded
- 1 tbsp. Parsley; chopped.
- 1 tbsp. Tomato sauce
- Salt and black pepper to taste.

Directions:

1.In a pan that fits your air fryer, mix the cabbage the rest of the ingredients except the parsley, toss, put the pan in the fryer and cook at 360°f for 15 minutes

2.Divide between plates and serve with parsley sprinkled on top.

Nutrition:

Calories: 163 kcal/Cal
Fat: 4 g
Fiber: 3 g
Carbohydrates: 6 g
Protein: 7 g

145.Pecan Brownies

Preparation Time: 30 minutes
Cooking Time: 20 minutes
Servings: 6
Ingredients:

- ¼ cup chopped pecans
- ¼ cup low carb
- Sugar: -free chocolate chips.
- ¼ cup unsalted butter; softened.
- 1 large egg.
- ½ cup blanched finely ground almond flour.
- ½ cup powdered erythritol
- 1 tbsp. Unsweetened cocoa powder
- ½ tsp. Baking powder.

Directions:

1.Take a large bowl, mix almond flour, erythritol, cocoa powder, and baking powder. Stir in butter and egg.

2.Adjust the temperature to 300°F and set the timer for 20 minutes. When fully cooked a toothpick inserted in the center will come out clean. Allow 20 minutes to fully cool and firm up.

Nutrition:

Calories: 215 kcal/Cal
Protein: 4.2 g
Fiber: 2.8 g
Fat: 18.9 g
Carbohydrates: 21.8 g

146.Cheesy Endives

Preparation Time: 20 minutes
Cooking Time: 15 minutes
Servings: 4
Ingredients:

- endives, trimmed
- ¼ cup goat cheese, crumbled
- 1 tbsp. Lemon juice
- 1 tbsp. Chives; chopped.
- 1 tbsp. Olive oil
- 1 tsp. Lemon zest, grated
- A pinch of salt and black pepper

Directions:

1.Take a bowl and mix the endives with the other ingredients except for the cheese and chives and toss well.

2.Put the endives in your air fryer's basket and cook at 380°F for 15 minutes

3.Divide the corn between plates.

4.Serve with cheese and chives sprinkled on top.

Nutrition:

Calories: 140 kcal/Cal
Fat: 4 g
Fiber: 3 g
Carbohydrates: 5 g
Protein: 7 g

147.Cauliflower Steak

Preparation Time: 12 minutes

Cooking Time: 7 minutes
Servings: 4
Ingredients:

- 1 medium head cauliflower
- ¼ cup blue cheese crumbles
- ¼ cup hot sauce
- ¼ cup full-fat ranch dressing
- 1 tbsp. Salted butter; melted.

Directions:
1.Remove cauliflower leaves. Slice the head in ½-inch-thick slices.
2.In a small bowl, mix hot sauce and butter. Brush the mixture over the cauliflower.
3.Place each cauliflower steak into the air fryer, working in batches if necessary. Adjust the temperature to 400°F and set the timer for 7 minutes
4.When cooked, edges will begin turning dark and caramelized. To serve, sprinkle steaks with crumbled blue cheese. Drizzle with ranch dressing.
Nutrition:
Calories: 122 kcal/Cal
Protein: 4.9 g
Fiber: 3.0 g
Fat: 8.4 g
Carbohydrates: 7.7 g

148.Parmesan Broccoli and Asparagus

Preparation Time: 20 minutes
Cooking Time: 15 minutes
Servings: 4
Ingredients:

- ½ lb. asparagus, trimmed
- 1 broccoli head, florets separated
- Juice of 1 lime
- 1 tbsp. parmesan, grated
- 1 tbsp. olive oil
- Salt and black pepper to taste.

Directions:
1.Take a bowl and mix the asparagus with the broccoli and all the other ingredients except the parmesan, toss, transfer to your air fryer's basket and cook at 400°F for 15 minutes
2.Divide between plates, sprinkle the parmesan on top, and serve.
Nutrition:
Calories: 172 kcal/Cal
Fat: 5 g
Fiber: 2 g
Carbohydrates: 4 g
Protein: 9 g

149.Air Fryer Crunchy Cauliflower

Preparation Time: 20 minutes
Cooking Time: 15 minutes
Servings: 5
Ingredients:

- oz. cauliflower
- 1 tbsp. potato starch
- 1 tsp. olive oil
- Salt & pepper to taste

Directions:
1. Set the air fryer toaster oven to 400°F and preheat it for 3 minutes. Slice cauliflower into equal pieces and if you are using potato starch, then toss with the florets into a bowl.
2. Add some olive oil and mix to coat.
3. Use olive oil cooking spray for spraying the inside of the air fryer toaster oven basket, then add cauliflower.
4. Cook for eight minutes, then shake the basket and cook for another 5 minutes depending on your desired level of crisp. Sprinkle roasted cauliflower with fresh parsley, kosher salt, and your seasonings or sauce of your choice.

Nutrition:
Calories: 36 kcal/Cal
Fat: 1 g
Protein: 1 g
Carbs: 5 g
Fiber: 2 g

150.Air Fryer Veg Buffalo Cauliflower

Preparation Time: 20 minutes
Cooking Time: 15 minutes
Servings: 3
Ingredients:

- 1 medium head cauliflower
- 1 tsp. avocado oil
- 1 tbsp. red hot sauce
- 1 tbsp. nutritional yeast
- 1 1/2 tsp. maple syrup
- 1/4 tsp. sea salt
- 1 tbsp. cornstarch or arrowroot starch

Directions:

1.Set your air fryer toaster oven to 360°F. Place all the ingredients to bowl except cauliflower. Mix them to combine.
2.Put the cauliflower and mix to coat equally. Put half of your cauliflower to air fryer and cook for 15 minutes but keep shaking them until your get desired consistency.
3. Do the same for the cauliflower which is left except lower **Cooking Time:** to 10 minutes.
4.Keep the cauliflower tightly sealed in refrigerator for 3-4 days. For heating again add back to air fryer for 1-2 minutes until crispness.

Nutrition:
Calories: 248 kcal/Cal
Fat: 20g
Protein: 4g
Carbs: 13g
Fiber: 2g

151.Air Fryer Asparagus

Preparation Time: 5 minutes
Cooking Time: 13 minutes
Servings: 2
Ingredients:

- Nutritional yeast
- Olive oil nonstick spray
- One bunch of asparagus

Directions:
1.Wash asparagus and then trim off thick, woody ends.
2.Spray asparagus with olive oil spray and sprinkle with yeast.
3.Add the asparagus to the air fryer rack/basket in a singular layer. Set temperature to 360°F and set time to 8 minutes. Select START/STOP to begin.

Nutrition:
Calories: 17 kcal/Cal
Total Fat: 8 g
Total Carbs: 2 g
Protein: 9 g

152.Almond Flour Battered and Crisped Onion Rings

Preparation Time: 5 minutes
Cooking Time: 20 minutes
Servings: 3
Ingredients:

- ½ cup almond flour
- ¾ cup coconut milk
- 1 big white onion, sliced into rings
- 1 egg, beaten
- 1 tablespoon baking powder
- 1 tablespoon smoked paprika
- Salt and pepper to taste

Directions:
1.Preheat the air fryer oven for 5 minutes.
2.In a mixing bowl, mix the almond flour, baking powder, smoked paprika, salt, and pepper.
3.In another bowl, combine the eggs and coconut milk.
4.Soak the onion slices into the egg mixture.
5.Dredge the onion slices in the almond flour mixture.
6.Pour into the Oven rack/basket. Set temperature to 325°F and set time to 15 minutes. Select START/STOP to begin. Shake the fryer basket for even cooking.

Nutrition:
Calories: 217 kcal/Cal
Total Fat: 17 g
Total Carbs: 2 g
Fiber: 6 g
Protein: 5 g

153.Divided Balsamic Mustard Greens

Preparation Time: 17 minutes;
Cooking Time: 15 minutes
Servings: 4
Ingredients:

- mustard greens - 1 bunch, trimmed
- olive oil - 2 tablespoons
- chicken stock - ½ cup
- tomato puree - 2 tablespoons
- garlic cloves - 3, minced
- Salt and black pepper to taste
- balsamic vinegar - 1 tablespoon

Directions:
1.Mix all of the ingredients in a pan that fits right into your air fryer and toss well.
2.Move the pan to the fryer and cook at a temperature of 260 o F for 12 minutes.
3.Divide all of it into different plates, serve your meal, and enjoy!

Nutrition:
calories 151,
fat 2,
fiber 4,

carbs 14,
protein 4

154.Butter Endives Recipe

Preparation Time: 15 minutes;
Cooking Time: 15 minutes
Servings: 4
Ingredients:

- Endives - 4, trimmed and halved
- Salt and black pepper to taste
- lime juice - 1 tablespoon
- Butter - 1 tablespoon, melted

Directions:
1.Place the endives in your air fryer, then add the salt and pepper to taste, lemon juice, and butter.
2.Cook at a temperature of 360 o F for 10 minutes.
3.Cut into different plates and serve right away.
Nutrition:
calories 100,
fat 3,
fiber 4,
carbs 8,
protein 4

155.Endives with Bacon Mix

Preparation Time: 15 minutes;
Cooking Time: 15 minutes
Servings: 4
Ingredients:

- Endives - 4, trimmed and halved
- Salt and black pepper to taste
- olive oil - 1 tablespoon
- bacon - 2 tablespoons, cooked and crumbled
- nutmeg - ½ teaspoon, ground

Directions:
1.Place the endives in your air fryer's basket, then add the salt and pepper to taste as well as oil and nutmeg; ensure to toss gently.
2.Cook at a temperature of 360 o F for 10 minutes.
3.Cut the endives into different plates, then sprinkle the bacon as toppings, and serve.
Nutrition:
calories 151,
fat 6,
fiber 8,
carbs 14,
protein 6

156.Sweet Beets Salad

Preparation Time: 20 Minutes
Cooking Time: 15 minutes
Servings: 4
Ingredients:

- Beets; peeled and quartered-1 ½-pound
- Brown sugar-2 tbsps
- Scallions; chopped-2
- Cider vinegar-2 tbsps
- Orange juice-1/2 cup
- Arugula-2 cups
- Mustard-2 tsps
- Olive oil- a drizzle
- Orange zest; grated-2 tsps

Directions:
1.Season the beets with orange juice and oil in a bowl.
2.Spread the beets in the air fryer basket and seal the fryer.
3.Cook the beets for 10 minutes at 3500 F on Air fryer mode.
4.Place these cooked beets in a bowl, then toss in orange zest, arugula, and scallions.
5.Whisk mustard, vinegar, and sugar in a different bowl.
6.Add this mixture to the beets and mix well.
7.Enjoy.
Nutrition:
calories 151,
fat 2,
fiber 4,
carbs 14,
protein 4

Chapter 16.Vegetables 2

157.Cheesy Cauliflower Fritters

Preparation Time: 5 minutes
Cooking Time: 14 minutes
Servings: 8
Ingredients:

- ½ C. chopped parsley
- 1 C. Italian breadcrumbs
- 1/3 C. shredded mozzarella cheese
- 1/3 C. shredded sharp cheddar cheese
- 1 egg
- minced garlic cloves
- chopped scallions
- 1 head of cauliflower

Directions:
1.Cut the cauliflower up into florets. Wash well and pat dry. Place into a food processor and pulse 20-30 seconds till it looks like rice.
2.Place the cauliflower rice in a bowl and mix with pepper, salt, egg, cheeses, breadcrumbs, garlic, and scallions.
3.With hands, form 15 patties of the mixture. Add more breadcrumbs if needed.
4.With olive oil, spritz patties, and place into your air fryer in a single layer.
5.Cook 14 minutes at 390 degrees, flipping after 7 minutes.
Nutrition:
Calories: 209
Fat: 17g
Protein: 6g
Sugar: 0.5g

158.Avocado Fries

Preparation Time: 5 minutes
Cooking Time: 5 minutes
Servings: 6
Ingredients:

- 1 avocado
- ½ tsp. salt
- ½ C. panko breadcrumbs
- Bean liquid (aquafaba) from a 15-ounce can of white or garbanzo beans

Directions:
1.Peel, pit, and slice up the avocado.
2.Toss salt and breadcrumbs together in a bowl. Place aquafaba into another bowl.
3.Dredge slices of avocado first in aquafaba and then in panko, making sure you get an even coating.
4.Place coated avocado slices into a single layer in the air fryer.
5.Cook 5 minutes at 390 degrees, shaking at 5 minutes.
6.Serve with your favorite dipping sauce!
Nutrition:
Calories: 102
Fat: 22g
Protein: 9g
Sugar: 1g

159.Zucchini Parmesan Chips

Preparation Time: 5 minutes
Cooking Time: 8 minutes
Servings: 10
Ingredients:

- ½ tsp. paprika
- ½ C. grated parmesan cheese
- ½ C. Italian breadcrumbs
- 1 lightly beaten egg
- thinly sliced zucchinis

Directions:
1.Use a very sharp knife or mandolin slicer to slice zucchini as thinly as you can. Pat off extra moisture.
2.Beat egg with a pinch of pepper and salt and a bit of water.
3.Combine paprika, cheese, and breadcrumbs in a bowl.
4.Dip slices of zucchini into the egg mixture and then into breadcrumb mixture. Press gently to coat.
5.With olive oil cooking spray, mist coated zucchini slices. Place into your air fryer in a single layer.
6.Cook 8 minutes at 350 degrees.
7.Sprinkle with salt and serve with salsa.
Nutrition:
Calories: 211
Fat: 16g
Protein: 8g
Sugar: 0g

160.Crispy Roasted Broccoli

Preparation Time: 45 minutes
Cooking Time: 15 minutes

Servings: 2
Ingredients:

- ¼ tsp. Masala
- ½ tsp. red chili powder
- ½ tsp. salt
- ¼ tsp. turmeric powder
- 1 tbsp. chickpea flour
- 1 tbsp. yogurt
- 1-pound broccoli

Directions:
1.Cut broccoli up into florets. Soak in a bowl of water with 2 teaspoons of salt for at least half an hour to remove impurities.
2.Take out broccoli florets from water and let drain. Wipe down thoroughly.
3.Mix all other ingredients together to create a marinade.
4.Toss broccoli florets in the marinade. Cover and chill 15-30 minutes.
5.Preheat air fryer to 390 degrees. Place marinated broccoli florets into the fryer. Cook 10 minutes.
6.minutes into cooking shake the basket. Florets will be crispy when done.
Nutrition:
Calories: 96
Fat: 1.3g
Protein: 7g
Sugar: 4.5g

161.Crispy Jalapeno Coins

Preparation Time: 10 minutes
Cooking Time: 10 minutes
Servings: 8 to 10
Ingredients:

- 1 egg
- 2-3 tbsp. coconut flour
- 1 sliced and seeded jalapeno
- Pinch of garlic powder
- Pinch of onion powder
- Pinch of Cajun seasoning (optional)
- Pinch of pepper and salt

Directions:
1.Ensure your air fryer is preheated to 400 degrees.
2.Mix together all dry ingredients.
3.Pat jalapeno slices dry. Dip coins into egg wash and then into dry mixture. Toss to thoroughly coat.
4.Add coated jalapeno slices to air fryer in a singular layer. Spray with olive oil.
5.Cook just till crispy.
Nutrition:
Calories: 128
Fat: 8g
Protein: 7g
Sugar: 0g

162.Buffalo Cauliflower

Preparation Time: 15 minutes
Cooking Time: 14 to 17 minutes
Servings: 6 to 8
Ingredients:
Cauliflower:

- 1 C. panko breadcrumbs
- 1 tsp. salt
- C. cauliflower florets

Buffalo Coating:

- ¼ C. Vegan Buffalo sauce
- ¼ C. melted vegan butter

Directions:
1.Melt butter in microwave and whisk in buffalo sauce.
2.Dip each cauliflower floret into buffalo mixture, ensuring it gets coated well. Hold over a bowl till floret is done dripping.
3.Mix breadcrumbs with salt.
4.Dredge dipped florets into breadcrumbs and place into the air fryer.
5.Cook 14-17 minutes at 350 degrees. When slightly browned, they are ready to eat!
6.Serve with your favorite keto dipping sauce!
Nutrition:
Calories: 194
Fat: 17g
Protein: 10g
Sugar: 3g

163.Jicama Fries

Preparation Time: 10 minutes
Cooking Time: 20 minutes
Servings: 8
Ingredients:

- 1 tbsp. dried thyme
- ¾ C. arrowroot flour
- ½ large Jicama
- 4 eggs

Directions:
1.Sliced jicama into fries.
2.Whisk eggs together and pour over fries. Toss to coat.

3.Mix a pinch of salt, thyme, and arrowroot flour together. Toss egg-coated jicama into dry mixture, tossing to coat well.
4.Spray air fryer basket with olive oil and add fries. Cook 20 minutes on CHIPS setting. Toss halfway into the cooking process.
Nutrition:
Calories: 211
Fat: 19g
Protein: 9g Sugar: 1g

164.Air Fryer Brussels Sprouts

Preparation Time: 5 minutes
Cooking Time: 10 minutes
Servings: 5
Ingredients:

- ¼ tsp. salt
- 1 tbsp. balsamic vinegar
- 1 tbsp. olive oil
- C. Brussels sprouts

Directions:
1.Cut Brussels sprouts in half lengthwise. Toss with salt, vinegar, and olive oil till coated thoroughly.
2.Add coated sprouts to the air fryer, cooking 8-10 minutes at 400 degrees. Shake after 5 minutes of cooking.
3.Brussels sprouts are ready to devour when brown and crisp!
Nutrition:
Calories: 118
Fat: 9g
Protein: 11g
Sugar: 1g

165.Spaghetti Squash Tots

Preparation Time: 5 minutes
Cooking Time: 15 minutes
Servings: 8 to 10
Ingredients:

- ¼ tsp. pepper
- ½ tsp. salt
- 1 thinly sliced scallion
- 1 spaghetti squash

Directions:
1.Wash and cut the squash in half lengthwise. Scrape out the seeds.
2.With a fork, remove spaghetti meat by strands and throw out skins.
3.In a clean towel, toss in squash and wring out as much moisture as possible. Place in a bowl and with a knife slice the meat a few times to cut up smaller.
4.Add pepper, salt, and scallions to squash and mix well.
5.Create "tot" shapes with your hands and place in the air fryer. Spray with olive oil.
6.Cook 15 minutes at 350 degrees until golden and crispy!
Nutrition:
Calories: 231
Fat: 18g
Protein: 5g
Sugar: 0g

166.Cinnamon Butternut Squash Fries

Preparation Time: 10 minutes
Cooking Time: 10 minutes
Servings: 2
Ingredients:

- 1 pinch of salt
- 1 tbsp. powdered unprocessed sugar
- ½ tsp. nutmeg
- 1 tsp. cinnamon
- 1 tbsp. coconut oil
- ounces pre-cut butternut squash fries

Directions:
1.In a plastic bag, pour in all ingredients. Coat fries with other components till coated and sugar is dissolved.
2.Spread coated fries into a single layer in the air fryer. Cook 10 minutes at 390 degrees until crispy.
Nutrition:
Calories: 175
Fat: 8g
Protein: 1g
Sugar: 5g

167.Carrot & Zucchini Muffins

Preparation Time: 5 minutes
Cooking Time: 14 minutes
Servings: 4
Ingredients:

- 2 tablespoons butter, melted
- ¼ cup carrots, shredded
- ½ cup zucchini, shredded
- 1 ½ cups almond flour
- 1 tablespoon liquid Stevia
- 2 teaspoons baking powder

- Pinch of salt
- 4 eggs
- 1 tablespoon yogurt
- 1 cup milk

Directions:

1.Preheat your air fryer to 350°Fahrenheit.
2.Beat the eggs, yogurt, milk, salt, pepper, baking soda, and Stevia.
3.Whisk in the flour gradually.
4.Add zucchini and carrots.
5.Grease muffin tins with butter and pour the muffin batter into tins. Cook for 14-minutes and serve.

Nutrition:

Calories: 224,
Total Fats: 12.3g,
Carbs: 11.2g,
Protein: 14.2g

168.Curried Cauliflower Florets

Preparation Time: 5 minutes
Cooking Time: 10 minutes
Servings: 4
Ingredients:

- 1/4 cup sultanas or golden raisins
- ¼ teaspoon salt
- 1 tablespoon curry powder
- 1 head cauliflower, broken into small florets
- ¼ cup pine nuts
- ½ cup olive oil

Directions:

1. In a cup of boiling water, soak your sultanas to plump. Preheat your air fryer to 350°Fahrenheit.
2. Add oil and pine nuts to the air fryer and toast for a minute or so.
3. In a bowl, toss the cauliflower and curry powder as well as salt, then add the mix to the air fryer mixing well.
4. Cook for 10-minutes. Drain the sultanas, toss with cauliflower, and serve.

Nutrition:

Calories: 275,
Total Fat: 11.3g,
Carbs: 8.6g,
Protein: 9.5g

169.Crispy Rye Bread Snacks with Guacamole and Anchovies

Preparation Time: 10 minutes
Cooking Time: 10 minutes
Servings: 4
Ingredients:

- slices of rye bread
- Guacamole
- Anchovies in oil

Directions:

1.Cut each slice of bread into 3 strips of bread.
2.Place in the basket of the air fryer without piling up, and we go in batches giving it the touch you want to give it. You can select 3500F, 10 minutes.
3.When you have all the crusty rye bread strips, put a layer of guacamole on top, whether homemade or commercial.
4.In each bread, place 2 anchovies on the guacamole.

Nutrition:

Calories: 180
Fat: 11.6g
Carbohydrates: 16g
Protein: 6.2g
Sugar: 0g
Cholesterol: 19.6mg

170.Oat and Chia Porridge

Preparation Time: 5 minutes
Cooking Time: 5 minutes
Servings: 4
Ingredients:

- 2 tablespoons peanut butter
- 2 teaspoons liquid Stevia
- 1 tablespoon butter, melted
- 2 cups milk
- 2 cups oats
- 1 cup chia seeds

Directions:

1.Preheat your air fryer to 390°Fahrenheit.
2.Whisk the peanut butter, butter, milk, and Stevia in a bowl.
3.Stir in the oats and chia seeds.
4.Pour the mixture into an oven-proof bowl and place in the air fryer, and cook for 5-minutes.

Nutrition:

Calories: 228,
Total Fats: 11.4g,
Carbs: 10.2g,
Protein: 14.5g

171.Feta & Mushroom Frittata

Preparation Time: 15 minutes
Cooking Time: 30 minutes
Servings: 4
Ingredients:

- 1 red onion, thinly sliced
- 2 cups button mushrooms, thinly sliced
- Salt to taste
- 2 tablespoons feta cheese, crumbled
- 4 medium eggs
- Non-stick cooking spray
- 2 tablespoons olive oil

Directions:

1.Sautė the onion and mushrooms in olive oil over medium heat until the vegetables are tender.
2. Remove the vegetables from the pan and drain on a paper towel-lined plate.
3. In a mixing bowl, whisk eggs and salt. Coat all sides of the baking dish with cooking spray.
4. Preheat your air fryer to 325°Fahrenheit. Pour the beaten eggs into the prepared baking dish and scatter the sautéed vegetables and crumble feta on top. Bake in the air fryer for 30-minutes. Allow to cool slightly and serve!

Nutrition:

Calories: 226,
Total Fat: 9.3g,
Carbs: 8.7g,
Protein: 12.6g

Chapter 17.Beef

172.Saucy Beef Bake

Preparation Time: 10 minutes
Cooking Time: 36 minutes
Servings: 6
Ingredients

- 2 tablespoons olive oil
- 1 large onion, diced
- lbs. (907.185g) Ground beef
- teaspoons salt
- cloves garlic, chopped
- 1/2 cup red wine
- cloves garlic, chopped
- 2 teaspoons ground cinnamon
- 2 teaspoons ground cumin
- 2 teaspoons dried oregano
- 1 teaspoon black pepper
- 1 can 28 oz. Crushed tomatoes
- 1 tablespoon tomato paste

Directions:

1.Put a suitable wok over moderate heat and add oil to heat.
2.Toss in onion, salt, and beef meat, then stir cook for 12 minutes.
3.Stir in red wine and cook for 2 minutes.
4.Add cinnamon, garlic, oregano, cumin, and pepper, then stir cook for 2 minutes.
5.Add tomato paste and tomatoes and cook for 20 minutes on a simmer.
6.Spread this mixture in a casserole dish.
7.Press the "power button" of the air fry oven and turn the dial to select the "bake" mode.
8.Press the time button and again turn the dial to set the cooking time to 30 minutes.
9.Now push the temp button and rotate the dial to set the temperature at 350 degrees f.
10. Once preheated, place the casserole dish in the oven and close its lid.
11. Serve warm.

Nutrition:

Calories 405
Total fat 22.7 g
Saturated fat 6.1 g
Cholesterol 4 mg
Sodium 227 mg
Total carbs 26.1 g
Fiber 1.4 g
Sugar 0.9 g
Protein 45.2 g

173.Parmesan Meatballs

Preparation Time: 10 minutes
Cooking Time: 20 minutes
Servings: 6
Ingredients

- lbs. (907.185g) Ground beef
- eggs
- 1 cup ricotta cheese
- 1/4 cup parmesan cheese shredded
- 1/2 cup panko breadcrumbs
- 1/4 cup basil chopped
- 1/4 cup parsley chopped
- 1 tablespoon fresh oregano chopped
- teaspoon kosher salt
- 1 teaspoon ground fennel
- 1/2 teaspoon red pepper flakes
- 32 oz spaghetti sauce, to serve

Directions:

1.Thoroughly mix the beef with all other ingredients for meatballs in a bowl.
2.Make small meatballs out of this mixture, then place them in the air fryer basket.
3.Press the "power button" of the air fry oven and turn the dial to select the "bake" mode.
4.Press the time button and again turn the dial to set the cooking time to 20 minutes.
5.Now push the temp button and rotate the dial to set the temperature at 400 degrees f.
6.Once preheated, place the meatballs basket in the oven and close its lid.
7.Flip the meatballs when cooked halfway through, then resume cooking.
8.Pour spaghetti sauce on top.
9.Serve warm.

Nutrition:

Calories 545
Total fat 36.4 g
Saturated fat 10.1 g
Protein 42.5 g

174.Tricolor Beef Skewers

Preparation Time: 10 minutes
Cooking Time: 25 minutes
Servings: 4
Ingredients

- garlic cloves, minced
- tablespoon rapeseed oil
- 1 cup cottage cheese, cubed

- cherry tomatoes
- tablespoon cider vinegar
- Large bunch thyme
- 1 ¼ lb. (566.99g) Boneless beef, diced

Directions:

- Toss beef with all its thyme, oil, vinegar, and garlic.
- Marinate the thyme beef for 2 hours in a closed container in the refrigerator.
- Thread the marinated beef, cheese, and tomatoes on the skewers.
- Place these skewers in an air fryer basket.
- Press the "power button" of the air fry oven and turn the dial to select the "air fry" mode.
- Press the time button and again turn the dial to set the cooking time to 25 minutes.
- Now push the temp button and rotate the dial to set the temperature at 350 degrees f.
- Once preheated, place the air fryer basket in the oven and close its lid.
- Flip the skewers when cooked halfway through, then resume cooking.
- Serve warm.

Nutrition:

Calories 695
Total fat 17.5 g
Saturated fat 4.8 g
Protein 117.4 g

175.Yogurt Beef Kebabs

Preparation Time: 10 minutes
Cooking Time: 25 minutes
Servings: 4
Ingredients

- ½ cup yogurt
- 1½ tablespoon mint
- 1 teaspoon ground cumin
- 1 cup eggplant, diced
- oz. Lean beef, diced
- ½ small onion, cubed

Directions:

1.Whisk yogurt with mint and cumin in a suitable bowl.
2.Toss in beef cubes and mix well to coat. Marinate for 30 minutes.
3.Alternatively, thread the beef, onion, and eggplant on the skewers.
4.Place these beef skewers in the air fry basket.
5.Press the "power button" of the air fry oven and turn the dial to select the "air fryer" mode.
6.Press the time button and again turn the dial to set the cooking time to 25 minutes.
7.Now push the temp button and rotate the dial to set the temperature at 370 degrees f.
8.Once preheated, place the air fryer basket in the oven and close its lid.
9.Flip the skewers when cooked halfway through, then resume cooking.
10. Serve warm.

Nutrition:

Calories 301
Total fat 8.9 g
Saturated fat 4.5 g
Protein 15.3 g

176.Agave Beef Kebabs

Preparation Time: 10 minutes
Cooking Time: 20 minutes
Servings: 6
Ingredients

- lbs. (907.185g) Beef steaks, cubed
- tablespoon jerk seasoning
- Zest and juice of 1 lime
- 1 tablespoon agave syrup
- ½ teaspoon thyme leaves, chopped

Directions:

1.Mix beef with jerk seasoning, lime juice, zest, agave and thyme.
2.Toss well to coat, then marinate for 30 minutes.
3.Alternatively, thread the beef on the skewers.
4.Place these beef skewers in the air fry basket.
5.Press the "power button" of the air fry oven and turn the dial to select the "air fryer" mode.
6.Press the time button and again turn the dial to set the cooking time to 20 minutes.
7.Now push the temp button and rotate the dial to set the temperature at 360 degrees f.
8.Once preheated, place the air fryer basket in the oven and close its lid.
9.Flip the skewers when cooked halfway through, then resume cooking.
10. Serve warm.

Nutrition:

Calories 548
Total fat 22.9 g
Saturated fat 9 g

Cholesterol 105 mg
Sodium 350 mg
Total carbs 17.5 g
Sugar 10.9 g
Fiber 6.3 g
Protein 40.1 g

177.Beef Skewers with Potato Salad

Preparation Time: 10 minutes
Cooking Time: 25 minutes
Servings: 4
Ingredients

- Juice ½ lemon
- 1 tablespoon olive oil
- 1 garlic clove, crushed
- 1 ¼ lb. (566.99g) Diced beef

For the salad

- potatoes, boiled, peeled and diced
- large tomatoes, chopped
- 1 cucumber, chopped
- 1 handful black olives, chopped
- oz. Pack feta cheese, crumbled
- 1 bunch of mint, chopped

Directions:

1.Whisk lemon juice with garlic and olive oil in a bowl.
2.Toss in beef cubes and mix well to coat. Marinate for 30 minutes.
3.Alternatively, thread the beef on the skewers.
4.Place these beef skewers in the air fry basket.
5.Press the "power button" of the air fry oven and turn the dial to select the "air fryer" mode.
6.Press the time button and again turn the dial to set the cooking time to 25 minutes.
7.Now push the temp button and rotate the dial to set the temperature at 360 degrees f.
8.Once preheated, place the air fryer basket in the oven and close its lid.
9.Flip the skewers when cooked halfway through, then resume cooking.
10. Meanwhile, whisk all the salad ingredients in a salad bowl.
11. Serve the skewers with prepared salad.

Nutrition:

Calories 609
Total fat 50.5 g
Saturated fat 11.7 g
Cholesterol 58 mg
Sodium 463 mg
Total carbs 9.9 g
Fiber 1.5 g
Sugar 0.3 g
Protein 29.3 g

178.Classic Souvlaki Kebobs

Preparation Time: 10 minutes
Cooking Time: 20 minutes
Servings: 6
Ingredients

- lbs. (907.185g) Beef shoulder fat trimmed, cut into chunks
- 1/3 cup olive oil
- ½ cup red wine
- 1 teaspoon dried oregano
- ½ cup of orange juice
- 1 teaspoon orange zest
- garlic cloves, crushed

Directions:

1.Whisk olive oil, red wine, oregano, oranges juice, zest, and garlic in a suitable bowl.
2.Toss in beef cubes and mix well to coat. Marinate for 30 minutes.
3.Alternatively, thread the beef, onion, and bread on the skewers.
4.Place these beef skewers in the air fry basket.
5.Press the "power button" of the air fry oven and turn the dial to select the "air fryer" mode.
6.Press the time button and again turn the dial to set the cooking time to 20 minutes.
7.Now push the temp button and rotate the dial to set the temperature at 370 degrees f.
8.Once preheated, place the air fryer basket in the oven and close its lid.
9.Flip the skewers when cooked halfway through, then resume cooking.
10. Serve warm.

Nutrition:

Calories 537
Total fat 19.8 g
Saturated fat 1.4 g
Cholesterol 10 mg
Sodium 719 mg
Total carbs 25.1 g
Fiber 0.9 g
Sugar 1.4 g
Protein 37.8 g

179.Harissa Dipped Beef Skewers

Preparation Time: 10 minutes
Cooking Time: 16 minutes
Servings: 6
Ingredients

- 1 lb. (453.592g) Beef mince
- 1 tablespoon harissa
- oz. Feta cheese
- 1 large red onion, shredded
- 1 handful parsley, chopped
- 1 handful mint, chopped
- 1 tablespoon olive oil

- Juice 1 lemon

Directions:

1.Whisk beef mince with harissa, onion, feta, and seasoning in a bowl.
2.Make 12 sausages out of this mixture, then thread them on the skewers.
3.Place these beef skewers in the air fry basket.
4.Press the "power button" of the air fry oven and turn the dial to select the "bake" mode.
5.Press the time button and again turn the dial to set the cooking time to 16 minutes.
6.Now push the temp button and rotate the dial to set the temperature at 370 degrees f.
7.Once preheated, place the air fryer basket in the oven and close its lid.
8.Flip the skewers when cooked halfway through, then resume cooking.
9.Toss the remaining salad ingredients in a salad bowl.
10. Serve beef skewers with tomato salad.

Nutrition:

Calories 452
Total fat 4 g
Saturated fat 2 g
Cholesterol 65 mg

180.Onion Pepper Beef Kebobs

Preparation Time: 10 minutes
Cooking Time: 20 minutes
Servings: 4

Ingredients

- 1 tablespoon pesto paste
- 2/3 lb. (303.9g) Beefsteak, diced
- red peppers, cut into chunks
- red onions, cut into wedges
- 1 tablespoon olive oil

Directions:

1.Toss in beef cubes with harissa and oil, then mix well to coat. Marinate for 30 minutes.
2.Alternatively, thread the beef, onion, and peppers on the skewers.
3.Place these beef skewers in the air fry basket.
4.Press the "power button" of the air fry oven and turn the dial to select the "air fryer" mode.
5.Press the time button and again turn the dial to set the cooking time to 20 minutes.
6.Now push the temp button and rotate the dial to set the temperature at 370 degrees f.
7.Once preheated, place the air fryer basket in the oven and close its lid.
8.Flip the skewers when cooked halfway through, then resume cooking.
9.Serve warm.

Nutrition:

Calories 301
Total fat 15.8 g
Saturated fat 2.7 g
Cholesterol 75 mg

181.Mayo Spiced Kebobs

Preparation Time: 10 minutes
Cooking Time: 10 minutes
Servings: 4

Ingredients

- 1 tablespoon cumin seed
- 1 tablespoon coriander seed
- 1 tablespoon fennel seed
- 1 tablespoon paprika
- 1 tablespoon garlic mayonnaise
- garlic cloves, finely minced
- ½ teaspoon ground cinnamon
- 1 ½ lb. (680.389g) Lean minced beef

Directions:

1.Blend all the spices and seeds with garlic, cream, and cinnamon in a blender.
2.Add this cream paste to the minced beef then mix well.
3.Make 8 sausages and thread each on the skewers.
4.Place these beef skewers in the air fry basket.
5.Press the "power button" of the air fry oven and turn the dial to select the "air fryer" mode.
6.Press the time button and again turn the dial to set the cooking time to 10 minutes.
7.Now push the temp button and rotate the dial to set the temperature at 370 degrees f.
8.Once preheated, place the air fryer basket in the oven and close its lid.
9.Flip the skewers when cooked halfway through, then resume cooking.
10. Serve warm.

Nutrition:

Calories 308
Total fat 20.5 g
Saturated fat 3 g
Cholesterol 42 mg

Chapter 18.Beef 2

182.Beef with Orzo Salad

Preparation Time: 10 minutes
Cooking Time: 27 minutes
Servings: 4
Ingredients

- 2/3 lbs. Beef shoulder, cubed
- 1 teaspoon ground cumin
- ½ teaspoon cayenne pepper
- 1 teaspoon sweet smoked paprika
- 1 tablespoon olive oil
- 24 cherry tomatoes

Salad:

- ½ cup orzo, boiled
- ½ cup frozen pea
- 1 large carrot, grated
- Small pack coriander, chopped
- Small pack mint, chopped
- Juice 1 lemon
- tablespoon olive oil

Directions:

1.Toss tomatoes and beef with oil, paprika, pepper, and cumin in a bowl.
2.Alternatively, thread the beef and tomatoes on the skewers.
3.Place these beef skewers in the air fry basket.
4.Press the "power button" of the air fry oven and turn the dial to select the "air fryer" mode.
5.Press the time button and again turn the dial to set the cooking time to 25 minutes.
6.Now push the temp button and rotate the dial to set the temperature at 370 degrees f.
7.Once preheated, place the air fryer basket in the oven and close its lid.
8.Flip the skewers when cooked halfway through, then resume cooking.
9.Meanwhile, sauté carrots and peas with olive oil in a pan for 2 minutes.
10. Stir in mint, lemon juice, coriander, and cooked couscous.
11. Serve skewers with the couscous salad.

Nutrition:

Calories 231
Total fat 20.1 g
Saturated fat 2.4 g
Cholesterol 110 mg
Sodium 941 mg
Total carbs 20.1 g
Fiber 0.9 g
Sugar 1.4 g
Protein 14.6 g

183.Beef Zucchini Shashliks

Preparation Time: 10 minutes
Cooking Time: 25 minutes
Servings: 4
Ingredients

- 1lb. (453.592g) Beef, boned and diced
- 1 lime, juiced and chopped
- tablespoon olive oil
- 20 garlic cloves, chopped
- 1 handful rosemary, chopped
- green peppers, cubed
- zucchinis, cubed
- red onions, cut into wedges

Directions:

1.Toss the beef with the rest of the skewer's ingredients in a bowl.
2.Thread the beef, peppers, zucchini, and onion on the skewers.
3.Place these beef skewers in the air fry basket.
4.Press the "power button" of the air fry oven and turn the dial to select the "air fryer" mode.
5.Press the time button and again turn the dial to set the cooking time to 25 minutes.
6.Now push the temp button and rotate the dial to set the temperature at 370 degrees f.
7.Once preheated, place the air fryer basket in the oven and close its lid.
8.Flip the skewers when cooked halfway through, then resume cooking.
9.Serve warm.

Nutrition:

Calories 472
Total fat 11.1 g
Saturated fat 5.8 g
Cholesterol 610 mg
Sodium 749 mg
Total carbs 19.9 g
Fiber 0.2 g
Sugar 0.2 g
Protein 13.5 g

184.Spiced Beef Skewers

Preparation Time: 10 minutes
Cooking Time: 18 minutes
Servings: 4
Ingredients

- 2 teaspoons ground cumin
- 2 teaspoons ground coriander
- 1/4 teaspoon ground cinnamon
- 1/8 teaspoon ground smoked paprika
- 2 teaspoons lime zest
- 1/2 teaspoon salt
- 1/2 teaspoon black pepper
- 1 tablespoon lemon juice
- 2 teaspoons olive oil
- 1 1/2 lbs. Lean beef, cubed

Directions:

1.Toss beef with the rest of the skewer's ingredients in a bowl.
2.Thread the beef and veggies on the skewers alternately.
3.Place these beef skewers in the air fry basket.
4.Press the "power button" of the air fry oven and turn the dial to select the "air fryer" mode.
5.Press the time button and again turn the dial to set the cooking time to 18 minutes.
6.Now push the temp button and rotate the dial to set the temperature at 370 degrees f.
7.Once preheated, place the air fryer basket in the oven and close its lid.
8.Flip the skewers when cooked halfway through, then resume cooking.
9.Serve warm.

Nutrition:

Calories 327
Total fat 3.5 g
Saturated fat 0.5 g
Cholesterol 162 mg
Sodium 142 mg
Total carbs 33.6 g
Fiber 0.4 g
Sugar 0.5 g
Protein 24.5 g

185.Beef Sausage with Cucumber Sauce

Preparation Time: 10 minutes
Cooking Time: 15 minutes
Servings: 6
Ingredients

- Beef kabobs
- 1 lb. (453.592g) Ground beef
- 1/2 an onion, finely diced
- garlic cloves, finely minced
- 2 teaspoons cumin
- 2 teaspoons coriander
- 1 ½ teaspoons salt
- 2 tablespoons chopped mint

Yogurt sauce:

- 1 cup Greek yogurt
- 2 tablespoons cucumber, chopped
- garlic cloves, minced
- 1/4 teaspoon salt

Directions:

1.Toss beef with the rest of the kebob ingredients in a bowl.
2.Make 6 sausages out of this mince and thread them on the skewers.
3.Place these beef skewers in the air fry basket.
4.Press the "power button" of the air fry oven and turn the dial to select the "air fryer" mode.
5.Press the time button and again turn the dial to set the cooking time to 15 minutes.
6.Now push the temp button and rotate the dial to set the temperature at 370 degrees f.
7.Once preheated, place the air fryer basket in the oven and close its lid.
8.Flip the skewers when cooked halfway through, then resume cooking.
9.Meanwhile, prepare the cucumber sauce by whisking all its ingredients in a bowl.
10. Serve the skewers with cucumber sauce.

Nutrition:

Calories 353
Total fat 7.5 g
Saturated fat 1.1 g
Cholesterol 20 mg
Sodium 297 mg
Total carbs 10.4 g
Fiber 0.2 g
Sugar 0.1 g
Protein 13.1 g

186.Beef Eggplant Medley

Preparation Time: 10 minutes
Cooking Time: 20 minutes
Servings: 4
Ingredients

- cloves of garlic
- 1 teaspoon dried oregano
- Olive oil
- beef steaks, diced
- eggplant, cubed
- fresh bay leaves
- lemons, juiced
- A few sprigs parsley, chopped

Directions:

1.Toss beef with the rest of the skewer's ingredients in a bowl.
2.Thread the beef and veggies on the skewers alternately.
3.Place these beef skewers in the air fry basket.
4.Press the "power button" of the air fry oven and turn the dial to select the "air fryer" mode.
5.Press the time button and again turn the dial to set the cooking time to 20 minutes.
6.Now push the temp button and rotate the dial to set the temperature at 370 degrees f.
7.Once preheated, place the air fryer basket in the oven and close its lid.
8.Flip the skewers when cooked halfway through, then resume cooking.
9.Serve warm.

Nutrition:

Calories 248
Total fat 13 g
Saturated fat 7 g
Cholesterol 387 mg
Sodium 353 mg
Total carbs 1 g
Fiber 0.4 g
Sugar 1 g
Protein 29 g

187.Glazed Beef Kebobs

Preparation Time: 10 minutes
Cooking Time: 20 minutes
Servings: 6
Ingredients

- lb. (453.592g) Beef, cubed
- 1/2 cup olive oil
- 1 lemon, juice only
- cloves garlic, minced
- 1 onion, sliced
- 1 teaspoon oregano, dried
- 1/4 teaspoon dried thyme,
- 1 teaspoon salt
- 1/4 teaspoon black pepper
- 1 tablespoon parsley, chopped
- 1 cup Worcestershire sauce

Directions:

1.Toss beef with the rest of the kebab ingredients in a bowl.
2.Cover the beef and marinate it for 30 minutes.
3.Thread the beef and veggies on the skewers alternately.
4.Place these beef skewers in the air fry basket. Brush the skewers with the Worcestershire sauce.
5.Press the "power button" of the air fry oven and turn the dial to select the "air fryer" mode.
6.Press the time button and again turn the dial to set the cooking time to 20 minutes.
7.Now push the temp button and rotate the dial to set the temperature at 370 degrees f.
8.Once preheated, place the air fryer basket in the oven and close its lid.
9.Flip the skewers when cooked halfway through, then resume cooking.
10. Serve warm.

Nutrition:

Calories 457
Total fat 19.1 g
Saturated fat 11 g
Cholesterol 262 mg
Sodium 557 mg
Total carbs 18.9 g
Sugar 1.2 g
Fiber 1.7 g
Protein 32.5 g

188.Beef Kebobs with Cream Dip

Preparation Time: 10 minutes
Cooking Time: 20 minutes
Servings: 6
Ingredients

- Beef kebabs
- lbs. (453.592g) Beef, diced
- 1 large onion, squares
- Salt

For the dressing

- 1 tablespoon mayonnaise
- 1 tablespoon olive oil
- 2 tablespoons lemon juice
- 1 teaspoon yellow mustard
- 1/4 teaspoon salt

- 1/8 teaspoon black pepper

Directions:

1.Toss beef and onion with salt in a bowl to season them.
2.Thread the beef and onion on the skewers alternately.
3.Place these beef skewers in the air fry basket.
4.Press the "power button" of the air fry oven and turn the dial to select the "air fryer" mode.
5.Press the time button and again turn the dial to set the cooking time to 20 minutes.
6.Now push the temp button and rotate the dial to set the temperature at 370 degrees f.
7.Once preheated, place the air fryer basket in the oven and close its lid.
8.Flip the skewers when cooked halfway through, then resume cooking.
9.Prepare the cream dip by mixing its ingredients in a bowl.
10. Serve skewers with cream dip.

Nutrition:

Calories 392
Total fat 16.1 g
Saturated fat 2.3 g
Cholesterol 231 mg
Sodium 466 mg
Total carbs 3.9 g
Sugar 0.6 g
Fiber 0.9 g
Protein 48 g

189.Asian Beef Skewers

Preparation Time: 10 minutes
Cooking Time: 15 minutes
Servings: 4
Ingredients

- 2 tablespoons hoisin sauce
- 2 tablespoons sherry
- 1/4 cup soy sauce
- 1 teaspoon barbeque sauce
- green onions, chopped
- cloves garlic, minced
- 1 tablespoon minced fresh ginger root
- 1 1/2 lbs. (453.592g) Flank steak, cubed

Directions:

1.Toss steak cubes with sherry, all the sauces, and other ingredients in a bowl.
2.Marinate the saucy spiced skewers for 30 minutes.
3.Place these beef skewers in the air fry basket.
4.Press the "power button" of the air fry oven and turn the dial to select the "air fryer" mode.
5.Press the time button and again turn the dial to set the cooking time to 15 minutes.
6.Now push the temp button and rotate the dial to set the temperature at 350 degrees f.
7.Once preheated, place the air fryer basket in the oven and close its lid.
8.Flip the skewers when cooked halfway through, then resume cooking.
9.Serve warm.

Nutrition:

Calories 321
Total fat 7.4 g
Saturated fat 4.6 g
Cholesterol 105 mg

190.Korean BBQ Skewers

Preparation Time: 10 minutes
Cooking Time: 15 minutes
Servings: 4
Ingredients

- oz. Lean sirloin steaks, cubed
- 1 small onion, finely diced
- 1/3 cup low sodium soy sauce
- 1/3 cup brown sugar
- 1 tablespoon sesame seeds
- 2 teaspoons sesame oil
- cloves garlic, diced
- 1 tablespoon ginger, grated
- 1 teaspoon sriracha
- 2 tablespoons honey
- Salt and pepper

Directions:

1.Toss steak cubes with sauces and other ingredients in a bowl.
2.Marinate the saucy spiced skewers for 30 minutes.
3.Place these beef skewers in the air fry basket.
4.Press the "power button" of the air fry oven and turn the dial to select the "air fryer" mode.
5.Press the time button and again turn the dial to set the cooking time to 15 minutes.

6.Now push the temp button and rotate the dial to set the temperature at 350 degrees f.
7.Once preheated, place the air fryer basket in the oven and close its lid.
8.Flip the skewers when cooked halfway through, then resume cooking.
9.Serve warm.

Nutrition:

Calories 248
Total fat 15.7 g
Saturated fat 2.7 g
Cholesterol 75 mg

191.Pork Rinds

Preparation Time: 10 minutes
Cooking Time: 7 minutes
Servings: 8

Ingredients

- 1 teaspoon chili flakes
- ½ teaspoon salt
- ½ teaspoon ground black pepper
- 1-pound pork rinds
- 1 teaspoon olive oil

Directions:

1.Heat up the air fryer to 365 F.
2.Sprinkle the air fryer basket with the inside olive oil.
3.Then place the pork rinds on the tray of the fryer.
4.Sprinkle salt and chili flakes with pork rinds and black ground pepper.
5.Mix them gently. Balance them gently.
6.Cook the pork rinds for 7 minutes after that.
7.When the time is done, shake the pork carefully.
8.Move the platter to the broad serving plate and allow 1-2 minutes to chill.
9.Serve and eat!

Nutrition:

Calories 329,
Fat 20.8,
Fiber 0,
Carbs 0.1,
Protein 36.5

Chapter 19.Seafood

192.Sesame Shrimp

Preparation Time: 8 minutes
Cooking Time: 15 minutes
Servings: 4
Ingredients:

- 1 lb. shrimp; peeled and deveined
- 1 tbsp. olive oil
- 1 tbsp. sesame seeds, toasted
- ½ tsp. Italian seasoning
- A pinch of salt and black pepper

Directions

1.Take a bowl and mix the shrimp with the rest of the ingredients and toss well, put the shrimp in the air fryer's basket.
2.Cook at 370°F for 12 minutes, and divide into bowls and serve.

Nutrition:

Calories: 199 Cal
Total Fat: 11 g
Saturated Fat: 0 g
Cholesterol: 0 mg
Sodium: 0 mg
Total Carbs: 4 g
Fiber: 2 g
Sugar: 0 g
Protein: 11 g

193.Salmon and Cauliflower Rice

Preparation Time: 10 minutes
Cooking Time: 30 minutes
Servings: 4
Ingredients:

- salmon fillets; boneless
- ½ cup chicken stock
- 1 cup cauliflower, riced
- 1 tbsp. butter; melted
- 1 tsp. turmeric powder
- Salt and black pepper to taste

Directions

1.In a pan that fits your air fryer, mix the cauliflower rice with the other ingredients except for the salmon and toss
2.Arrange the salmon fillets over the cauliflower rice, put the pan in the fryer, and cook at 360°F for 25 minutes, flipping the fish after 15 minutes
3.Divide everything between plates and serve.

Nutrition:

Calories: 241 Cal
Total Fat: 12 g
Saturated Fat: 0 g
Cholesterol: 0 mg
Sodium: 0 mg
Total Carbs: 6 g
Fiber: 2 g
Sugar: 0 g
Protein: 12 g

194.Tilapia and Salsa

Preparation Time: 10 minutes
Cooking Time: 20 minutes
Servings: 4
Ingredients:

- tilapia fillets; boneless
- oz. canned tomatoes; chopped.
- 1 tbsp. green onions; chopped.
- 1 tbsp. sweet red pepper; chopped.
- 1 tbsp. balsamic vinegar
- 1 tbsp. olive oil
- A pinch of salt and black pepper

Directions:

1.Arrange the tilapia in a baking sheet that fits the air fryer and season with salt and pepper.
2.In a bowl, combine all the other ingredients, toss, and spread over the fish, introduce the pan in the fryer and cook at 350°F for 15 minutes
3.Divide the mix between plates and serve.

Nutrition:

Calories: 221 Cal
Total Fat: 12 g
Saturated Fat: 0 g
Cholesterol: 0 mg
Sodium: 0 mg
Total Carbs: 5 g
Fiber: 2 g
Sugar: 0 g
Protein: 14 g

195.Garlic Tilapia

Preparation Time: 10 minutes
Cooking Time: 25 minutes
Servings: 4
Ingredients:

- tilapia fillets; boneless
- 1 bunch kale; chopped.

- garlic cloves; minced
- 1 tbsp. olive oil
- 1 tsp. fennel seeds
- ½ tsp. red pepper flakes, crushed
- Salt and black pepper to taste

Directions

1.In a pan that fits the fryer, combine all the ingredients put the pan in the fryer and cook at 360°F for 20 minutes divide everything between plates and serve.

Nutrition:

Calories: 240 Cal
Total Fat: 12 g
Saturated Fat: 0 g
Cholesterol: 0 mg
Sodium: 0 mg
Total Carbs: 4 g
Fiber: 2 g
Sugar: 0 g
Protein: 12 g

196.Trout and Mint

Preparation Time: 10 minutes
Cooking Time: 21 minutes
Servings: 4
Ingredients:

- 1 avocado, peeled, pitted and roughly chopped.
- rainbow trout
- 1/3 pine nuts
- 1 cup olive oil + 3 tbsp.
- 1 cup parsley; chopped.
- garlic cloves; minced
- ½ cup mint; chopped.
- Zest of 1 lemon
- Juice of 1 lemon
- A pinch of salt and black pepper

Directions:

1 Pat dries the trout, season with salt and pepper, and rub with 3 tbsp. oil
2.Put the fish in your air fryer's basket and cook for 8 minutes on each side.
3.Divide the fish between plates and drizzle half of the lemon juice all over in a blender.
4.Combine the rest of the oil with the remaining lemon juice, parsley, garlic, mint, lemon zest, pine nuts, and the avocado and pulse well. Spread this over the trout and serve.

Nutrition:

Calories: 240 Cal
Total Fat: 12 g
Saturated Fat: 0 g
Cholesterol: 0 mg
Sodium: 0 mg
Total Carbs: 6 g
Fiber: 4 g
Sugar: 0 g
Protein: 9 g

197.Salmon and Coconut Sauce

Preparation Time: 25 minutes
Cooking Time: 10 minutes
Servings: 4
Ingredients:

- salmon fillets; boneless
- 1/3 cup heavy cream
- ¼ cup lime juice
- ½ cup coconut; shredded
- ¼ cup coconut cream
- 1 tsp. lime zest; grated
- A pinch of salt and black pepper

Directions:

1.Take a bowl and mix all the ingredients except the salmon and whisk.
2.Arrange the fish in a pan that fits your air fryer, drizzle the coconut sauce all over, put the pan in the machine, and cook at 360°F for 20 minutes. Divide between plates and serve

Nutrition:

Calories: 227 Cal
Total Fat: 12 g
Saturated Fat: 0 g
Cholesterol: 0 mg
Sodium: 0 mg
Total Carbs: 4 g
Fiber: 2 g
Sugar: 0 g
Protein: 9 g

198.Simple Salmon

Preparation Time: 10 minutes
Cooking Time: 22 minutes
Servings: 2
Ingredients:

- (4-oz. salmon fillets, skin removed
- 1 medium lemon
- 1 tbsp. unsalted butter; melted.
- ½ tsp. dried dill
- ½ tsp. garlic powder

Directions:

1.Place each fillet on a 5" × 5" square of aluminum foil. Drizzle with butter and sprinkle with garlic powder.
2.Zest half of the lemon and sprinkle zest over salmon. Slice other half of the lemon and lay two slices on each piece of salmon.
3.Sprinkle dill over salmon Gather and fold foil at the top and sides to fully close packets.
4.Place foil packets into the air fryer basket. Adjust the temperature to 400°F and set the timer for 12 minutes Salmon will be easily flaked and have an internal temperature of at least 145°F when fully cooked.

Nutrition:
Calories: 252 Cal
Total Fat: 15 g
Saturated Fat: 0 g
Cholesterol: 0 mg
Sodium: 0 mg
Total Carbs: 2 g
Fiber: 4 g
Sugar: 0 g
Protein: 29 g

199.Cajun Salmon

Preparation Time: 5 minutes
Cooking Time: 12 minutes
Servings: 2
Ingredients:

- (4-oz. salmon fillets, skin removed
- 1 tbsp. unsalted butter; melted.
- 1 tsp. paprika
- ¼ tsp. ground black pepper
- ⅛ Tsp. ground cayenne pepper
- ½ tsp. garlic powder

Directions:
1.Brush each fillet with butter.
2.Combine remaining ingredients in a small bowl and then rub onto fish. Place fillets into the air fryer basket, adjust the temperature to 390°F and set the timer for 7 minutes.
3.When fully cooked, the internal temperature will be 145°F. Serve right away.

Nutrition:
Calories: 253 Cal
Total Fat: 16 g
Saturated Fat: 0 g
Cholesterol: 0 mg
Sodium: 0 mg
Total Carbs: 4 g
Fiber: 4 g
Sugar: 0 g
Protein: 29 g

200.Salmon and Sauce

Preparation Time: 10 minutes
Cooking Time: 25 minutes
Servings: 4
Ingredients:

- salmon fillets; boneless
- garlic cloves; minced
- ¼ cup ghee; melted
- ½ cup heavy cream
- 1 tbsp. chives; chopped.
- 1 tsp. lemon juice
- 1 tsp. dill; chopped.

A pinch of salt and black pepper

Directions:
1.Take a bowl and mix all the ingredients except the salmon and whisk well.
2.Arrange the salmon in a pan that fits the air fryer, drizzle the sauce all over, introduce the pan in the machine, and cook at 360°F for 20 minutes. Divide everything between plates and serve

Nutrition:
Calories: 220 Cal
Total Fat: 14 g
Saturated Fat: 0 g
Cholesterol: 0 mg
Sodium: 0 mg
Total Carbs: 5 g
Fiber: 2 g
Sugar: 0 g
Protein: 12 g

201.Indian Fish Fingers

Preparation Time: 35 minutes
Cooking Time: 50 minutes
Servings: 4
Ingredients:

- 1/2-pound fish fillet
- 1 tablespoon finely chopped fresh mint leaves or any fresh herbs
- 1/3 cup breadcrumbs
- 1 teaspoon ginger garlic paste or ginger and garlic powders
- 1 hot green chili finely chopped
- 1/2 teaspoon paprika
- Generous pinch of black pepper
- Salt to taste
- 3/4 tablespoons lemon juice

- 3/4 teaspoons gram masala powder
- 1/3 teaspoon rosemary
- 1 egg

Directions:

1.Start by removing any skin on the fish, washing, and patting dry. Cut the fish into fingers.

2.In a medium bowl, mix together all ingredients except for fish, mint, and breadcrumbs. Bury the fingers in the mixture and refrigerate for 30 minutes.

3.Remove from the bowl from the fridge and mix in mint leaves.

4.In a separate bowl, beat the egg, pour breadcrumbs into a third bowl. Dip the fingers in the egg bowl, then toss them in the breadcrumbs bowl.

5.Pour into the oven rack/basket. Place the grill on the center shelf of the oven with the air fryer. Set the temperature to 360 ° F and set the time to 15 minutes. Move your fingers in half.

Nutrition:

Calories: 441 Cal
Total Fat: 38 g
Total Carbs: 2 g
Fiber: 6 g
Protein: 11 g

202.Healthy Fish and Chips

Preparation Time: 5 minutes
Cooking Time: 20 minutes
Servings: 3
Ingredients:

- Old Bay seasoning
- ½ C. panko breadcrumbs
- 1 egg
- 1 tbsp. almond flour
- 4-6-ounce tilapia fillets
- Frozen crinkle cut fries

Directions:

1.Add almond flour to one bowl, beat egg in another bowl, and add panko breadcrumbs to the third bowl, mixed with Old Bay seasoning.

2.Dredge tilapia in flour, then egg, and then breadcrumbs.

3.Place coated fish in the air fryer oven along with fries.

4.Set temperature to 390°F and set time to 15 minutes

Nutrition:

Calories: 219 Cal
Total Fat: 5 g
Total Carbs: 2 g
Fiber: 6 g
Protein: 25 g

.

203.Quick Paella

Preparation Time: 7 minutes
Cooking Time: 22 minutes
Servings: 4
Ingredients:

- 1 (10-ounce) package frozen cooked rice, thawed
- 1 (6-ounce) jar artichoke hearts, drained and chopped
- ¼ cup vegetable broth
- ½ teaspoon turmeric
- ½ teaspoon dried thyme
- 1 cup frozen cooked small shrimp
- ½ cup frozen baby peas
- 1 tomato, diced

Directions:

1.In a 6-by-6-by-2-inch pan, combine the rice, artichoke hearts, vegetable broth, turmeric, and thyme, and stir gently.

2.Place in the air fryer oven and bake for 8 to 9 minutes or until the rice is hot. Remove from the air fryer and gently stir in the shrimp, peas, and tomato. Cook for 5 to 8 minutes or until the shrimp and peas are hot, and the paella is bubbling.

Nutrition:

Calories: 345 Cal
Total Fat: 1g
Total Carbs: 2 g
Fiber: 6 g
Protein: 18 g

204.Coconut Shrimp

Preparation Time: 15 minutes
Cooking Time: 30 minutes
Servings: 10
Ingredients:

- 1 (8-ounce) can crushed pineapple
- ½ cup sour cream
- ¼ cup pineapple preserves
- 2 egg whites
- ⅔ Cup cornstarch
- ⅔ Cup sweetened coconut
- 1 cup panko breadcrumbs

- 1-pound uncooked large shrimp, thawed if frozen, deveined and shelled Olive oil for misting

Directions:

1.Drain the crushed pineapple well, reserving the juice.
2.In a small bowl, combine the pineapple, sour cream, and preserves, and mix well.
3. Set aside. In a shallow bowl, beat the egg whites with 2 tablespoons of the reserved pineapple liquid.
4. Place the cornstarch on a plate. Combine the coconut and breadcrumbs on another plate.
5.Dip the shrimp into the cornstarch, shake it off, then dip into the egg white mixture and finally into the coconut mixture.
6.Place the shrimp in the air fryer basket and mist with oil.
7.Cook for 5 to 7 minutes or until the shrimp are crisp and golden brown

Nutrition:

Calories: 441 Cal
Total Fat: 38 g
Total Carbs: 2 g
Fiber: 6 g
Protein: 18 g

205.3-Ingredient Air Fryer Catfish

Preparation Time: 5 minutes
Cooking Time: 20 minutes
Servings: 3

Ingredients:

- 1 tbsp. chopped parsley
- 1 tbsp. olive oil
- ¼ C. seasoned fish fry
- catfish fillets

Directions:

1.Ensure your air fryer oven is preheated to 400 °.
2.Rinse off catfish fillets and pat dry.
3.Add fish fry seasoning to Ziploc baggie, then catfish. Shake the bag and ensure the fish gets well coated.
4.Spray each fillet with olive oil.
5.Add fillets to the air fryer basket.
6.Set temperature to 400°F and set time to 10 minutes.
7.Cook 10 minutes. Then flip and cook another 2-3 minutes.

Nutrition:

Calories: 208 Cal
Total Fat: 38 g
Total Carbs: 2 g
Fiber: 6 g
Protein: 18 g

Chapter 20.Seafood 2

206.Scallops and Spring Veggies

Preparation Time: 10 minutes
Cooking Time: 8 minutes
Servings: 4
Ingredients

- ½ pound (226.8g) asparagus, ends trimmed, cut into 2-inch pieces
- 1 cup sugar snap peas
- 1-pound (453.592g) sea scallops
- 1 tablespoon lemon juice
- 2 teaspoons olive oil
- ½ teaspoon dried thyme
- Pinch salt
- Freshly ground black pepper

Directions:

1.Place the asparagus and sugar snap peas in the air fryer basket.
2.Cook for 2 to 3 minutes or until the vegetables are just starting to get tender.
3.Meanwhile, check the scallops for a small muscle attached to the side, and pull it off and discard.
4.In a medium bowl, toss the scallops with lemon juice, olive oil, thyme, salt, and pepper. Place into the air fryer oven basket on top of the vegetables.
5.Steam for 5 to 7 minutes, tossing the basket once during cooking time until the scallops are just firm when tested with your finger and are opaque in the center, and the vegetables are tender. Serve immediately.

Nutrition:

calories: 162;
carbs:10g;
fat: 4g;
protein:22g;
fiber:3g

207.Air Fryer Salmon Patties

Preparation Time: 8 minutes
Cooking Time: 7 minutes
Servings: 4
Ingredients

- 1 tbsp. Olive oil
- 1 tbsp. Ghee
- ¼ tsp. Salt
- 1/8 tsp. Pepper
- 1 egg
- 1 c. Almond flour
- 1 can wild Alaskan pink salmon

Directions:

1.Drain can of salmon into a bowl and keep liquid. Discard skin and bones.
2.Add salt, pepper, and egg to salmon, mixing well with hands to incorporate. Make patties.
3.Dredge in flour and remaining egg. If it seems dry, spoon reserved salmon liquid from the can onto patties.
4.Place the rack on the middle-shelf of the air fryer oven. Set temperature to 378°f, and set time to 7 minutes. Cook 7 minutes till golden, making sure to flip once during cooking process.

Nutrition:

calories: 437;
carbs:55;
fat: 12g;
protein:24g;
sugar:2g

208.Salmon Noodles

Preparation Time: 5 minutes
Cooking Time: 16 minutes
Servings: 4
Ingredients

- 1 salmon fillet
- 1 tbsp teriyaki marinade
- ½ ozs soba noodles, cooked and drained
- ozs firm tofu
- ozs mixed salad
- 1 cup broccoli
- Olive oil
- Salt and pepper to taste

Directions:

1.Season the salmon with salt and pepper to taste, then coat with the teriyaki marinade. Set aside for 15 minutes
2.Preheat the air fryer oven at 350 degrees, then cook the salmon for 8 minutes.
3.Whilst the air fryer is cooking the salmon, start slicing the tofu into small cubes.
4.Next, slice the broccoli into smaller chunks. Drizzle with olive oil.
5.Once the salmon is cooked, put the broccoli and tofu into the air fryer oven tray for 8 minutes.

6.Plate the salmon and broccoli tofu mixture over the soba noodles. Add the mixed salad to the side and serve.

Nutrition:

calories: 437;
carbs:55;
fat: 12g;
protein:24g;
sugar:2g

209.Beer-Battered Fish and Chips

Preparation Time: 5 minutes
Cooking Time: 30 minutes
Servings: 4

Ingredients

- 4 eggs
- 1 cup malty beer, such as pabst blue ribbon
- 1 cup all-purpose flour
- ½ cup cornstarch
- 1 teaspoon garlic powder
- Salt
- Pepper
- Cooking oil
- (4-ounce) cod fillets

Directions:

1.in a medium bowl, beat the eggs with the beer. In another medium bowl, combine the flour and cornstarch, and season with the garlic powder and salt and pepper to taste.
1.Spray the air fryer basket with cooking oil.
2.Dip each cod fillet in the flour and cornstarch mixture and then in the egg and beer mixture. Dip the cod in the flour and cornstarch a second time.
3.place the cod in the air fryer oven. Do not stack. Cook in batches. Spray with cooking oil. Cook for 8 minutes.
4.Open the air fryer oven and flip the cod. Cook for an additional 7 minutes.
5.Remove the cooked cod from the air fryer, then repeat steps 4 and 5 for the remaining fillets.
6.Serve with prepared air fried frozen fries. Frozen fries will need to be cooked for 18 to 20 minutes at 400ºf.
7.Cool before serving.

Nutrition:

calories: 325;
carbs:41;
fat: 4g;
protein:26g;
fiber:1g

210.Tuna Stuffed Potatoes

Preparation Time: 5 minutes
Cooking Time: 30 minutes
Servings: 4

Ingredients

- starchy potatoes
- ½ tablespoon olive oil
- 1 (6-ounce) can tuna, drained
- tablespoons plain greek yogurt
- 1 teaspoon red chili powder
- Salt and freshly ground black pepper to taste
- 1 scallion, chopped and divided
- 1 tablespoon capers

Directions:

1. In a large bowl of water, soak the potatoes for about 30 minutes. Drain well and pat dry with paper towel.
2. Preheat the air fryer to 355 degrees f. Place the potatoes in a fryer basket.
3. Cook for about 30 minutes.
4. Meanwhile in a bowl, add tuna, yogurt, red chili powder, salt, black pepper and half of scallion and with a potato masher, mash the mixture completely.
5. Remove the potatoes from the air fryer oven and place onto a smooth surface.
6. Carefully, cut each potato from top side lengthwise.
7. With your fingers, press the open side of potato halves slightly. Stuff the potato open portion with tuna mixture evenly.
8. Sprinkle with the capers and remaining scallion. Serve immediately.

Nutrition:

Calories: 795,
Protein: 109.77g,
Fat: g,
Carbs: g

211.Fried Calamari

Preparation Time: 8 minutes
Cooking Time: 7 minutes
Servings: 6-8

Ingredients

- ½ tsp. Salt
- ½ tsp. Old bay seasoning
- 1/3 c. Plain cornmeal

- ½ c. Semolina flour
- ½ c. Almond flour
- 5-6 c. Olive oil
- 1 ½ pound (680.389g) baby squid

Directions:

1. Rinse squid in cold water and slice tentacles, keeping just ¼-inch of the hood in one piece.
2. Combine 1-2 pinches of pepper, salt, old bay seasoning, cornmeal, and both flours together. Dredge squid pieces into flour mixture and place into the air fryer basket.
3. Spray liberally with olive oil. Cook 15 minutes at 345 degrees till coating turns a golden brown.

Nutrition:

calories: 211;
carbs:55;
fat: 6g;
protein:21g;
sugar:1g

212.Soy and Ginger Shrimp

Preparation Time: 8 minutes
Cooking Time: 10 minutes
Servings: 4
Ingredients

- 2 tablespoons olive oil
- 2 tablespoons scallions, finely chopped
- cloves garlic, chopped
- 1 teaspoon fresh ginger, grated
- 1 tablespoon dry white wine
- 1 tablespoon balsamic vinegar
- 1/4 cup soy sauce
- 1 tablespoon sugar
- 1 pound (453.592g) shrimp
- Salt and ground black pepper to taste

Directions:

1.To make the marinade, warm the oil in a saucepan; cook all ingredients, except the shrimp, salt, and black pepper. Now, let it cool.
2.Marinate the shrimp, covered, at least an hour, in the refrigerator.
3.After that, pour inside the oven rack/basket.
4.Set the rack on the middle shelf of the air fryer oven.
5.Set temperature to 350°f and set time to 10 minutes. Bake the shrimp at 350 degrees f for 8 to 10 minutes (depending on the size), turning once or twice.
6.Season prepared shrimp with salt and black pepper and serve.

Nutrition:

Calories: 233,
Protein: 24.55g,
Fat: 10.28g,
Carbs: 10.86g

213.Crispy Cheesy Fish Fingers

Preparation Time: 10 minutes
Cooking Time: 20 minutes
Servings: 4
Ingredients

- Large cod fish filet, approximately 6-8 ounces, fresh or frozen and thawed, cut into 1 ½-inch strips
- raw eggs
- ½ cup of breadcrumbs (we like panko, but any brand or home recipe will do)
- 2 tablespoons of shredded or powdered parmesan cheese
- 1 tablespoon of shredded cheddar cheese
- Pinch of salt and pepper

Directions:

1. Cover the basket of the air fryer oven with a lining of tin foil, leaving the edges uncovered to allow air to circulate through the basket.
2. Preheat the air fryer oven to 350 degrees.
3. In a large mixing bowl, beat the eggs until fluffy and until the yolks and whites are fully combined.
4. Dunk all the fish strips in the beaten eggs, fully submerging.
5. In a separate mixing bowl, combine the bread crumbs with the parmesan, cheddar, and salt and pepper, until evenly mixed.
6. One by one, coat the egg-covered fish strips in the mixed dry ingredients so that they're fully covered, and place on the foil-lined air fryer basket.
7. Set the air fryer oven timer to 20 minutes.
8. Halfway through the cooking time, shake the handle of the air fryer so that the

breaded fish jostles inside and fry coverage is even.

9. After 20 minutes, when the fryer shuts off, the fish strips will be perfectly cooked, and their breaded crust golden-brown and delicious! Using tongs, remove from the air fryer and set on a serving dish to cool.

Nutrition:

Calories: 124,

Protein: 6.86g,

Fat: 5.93g,

Carbs: 12.26g

214.Panko-Crusted Tilapia

Preparation Time: 5 minutes

Cooking Time: 10 minutes

Servings: 3

Ingredients

- 2 tsp. Italian seasoning
- 1 tsp. Lemon pepper
- 1/3 c. Panko breadcrumbs
- 1/3 c. Egg whites
- 1/3 c. Almond flour
- tilapia fillets
- Olive oil

Directions:

1 Place panko, egg whites, and flour into separate bowls. Mix lemon pepper and italian seasoning in with breadcrumbs.

2.Pat tilapia fillets dry. Dredge in flour, then egg, then breadcrumb mixture.

3.Add to the air fryer basket and spray lightly with olive oil.

4.Cook 10-11 minutes at 400 degrees, making sure to flip halfway through cooking.

Nutrition:

calories: 256;

fat: 9g;

protein:39g;

sugar:5g

215.Potato Crusted Salmon

Preparation Time: 10 minutes

Cooking Time: 15 minutes

Servings: 4

Ingredients

- 1 pound (453.592g) salmon, swordfish, or arctic char fillets, 3/4 inch thick
- 1 egg white
- 2 tablespoons water
- 1/3 cup dry instant mashed potatoes
- 2 teaspoons cornstarch
- 1 teaspoon paprika
- 1 teaspoon lemon pepper seasoning

Directions:

1.Remove and skin from the fish and cut it into 4 serving pieces, mix together the egg white and water. Mix together all of the dry ingredients. Dip the fillets into the egg white mixture, then press into the potato mix to coat evenly.

2.Pour on the oven shelf/basket. Place the grill in the center of the frame of the pots.

3.Set temperature to 360°f, and set time to 15 minutes, flip the filets halfway through.

Nutrition:

calories:176;

fat: 7g;

protein:23g;

216.Salmon Croquettes

Preparation Time: 5 minutes

Cooking Time: 10 minutes

Servings: 6-8

Ingredients

- Panko breadcrumbs
- Almond flour
- 4 egg whites
- 1 tbsp. Chopped chives
- 1 tbsp. Minced garlic cloves
- ½ c. Chopped onion
- 2/3 c. Grated carrots
- 1 pound (453.592g) chopped salmon fillet

Directions:

1.Mix together all ingredients minus breadcrumbs, flour, and egg whites.

2.Shape mixture into balls. Then coat them in flour, then egg, and then breadcrumbs. Drizzle with olive oil.

3.Pour the coated salmon balls into the oven rack/basket. Place the rack on the middle shelf of the air fryer oven. Set temperature to 350°f and set time to 6 minutes. Shake and cook an additional 4 minutes until golden in color.

Nutrition:

calories: 503;

carbs:61g;

fat: 9g;

protein:5g;

sugar:4g

217.Snapper Scampi

Preparation Time: 5 minutes
Cooking Time: 10 minutes
Servings: 4
Ingredients

- (6-ounce) skinless snapper or arctic char fillets
- 1 tablespoon olive oil
- 2 tablespoons lemon juice, divided
- ½ teaspoon dried basil
- Pinch salt
- Freshly ground black pepper
- 2 tablespoons butter
- Cloves garlic, minced

Directions:

1.Rub the fish fillets with olive oil and 1 tablespoon of lemon juice. Sprinkle with the basil, salt, and pepper, and place in the air fryer oven basket.
2.Grill the fish for 7 to 8 minutes or until the fish just flakes when tested with a fork.
3.Remove the fish from the basket and put on a serving plate. Cover to keep warm.
4.In a 6-by-6-by-2-inch pan, combine the butter, remaining 2 tablespoons lemon juice, and garlic.
5. Cook in the air fryer oven for 1 to 2 minutes or until the garlic is sizzling.
6.Pour this mixture over the fish and serve.

Nutrition:

calories: 265;
carbs:1g;
fat: 11g;
protein:39g;
fiber:0g

Chapter 21.Snacks

218.Sweet Potato Tater Tots

Preparation Time: 10 minutes.
Cooking Time: 23 minutes.
Servings: 4
Ingredients:

- sweet potatoes, peeled
- 1/2 tsp. Cajun seasoning
- Olive oil cooking spray
- Sea salt to taste

Directions:

1.Boil sweet potatoes in water for 15 minutes over medium-high heat.
2.Drain the sweet potatoes, then allow them to cool
3.Peel the boiled sweet potatoes and return them to the bowl.
4.Mash the potatoes and stir in salt and Cajun seasoning. Mix well and make small tater tots out of it.
5.Place the tater tots in the Air Fryer basket and spray them with cooking oil.
6.Place the Air Fryer basket inside the Air Fryer toaster and close the lid.
7.Select Air Frying mode at a temperature of 400 ° F for 8 minutes.
8.Turn the trays over and continue cooking for another 8 minutes.
9.Serve fresh.

Nutrition:
Calories: 184 Cal
Protein: 9 g
Carbs: 43 g
Fat: 17 g

219.Fried Ravioli

Preparation Time: 10 minutes
Cooking Time: 15 minutes
Servings: 4
Ingredients:

- 1 package ravioli, frozen
- 1 cup breadcrumbs
- 1/2 cup parmesan cheese
- 1 tbs. Italian seasoning
- 1 tbs. garlic powder
- eggs, beaten
- Cooking spray

Directions:

1.Mix breadcrumbs with garlic powder, cheese, and Italian seasoning in a bowl.
2.Whisk eggs in another bowl. Dip each ravioli in eggs first, then coat them with crumbs mixture.
3. Place the ravioli in the Air Fryer basket. Place the air Fryer basket inside the oven and close the lid.
4.Select the Air Fry mode at 360°F temperature for 15 minutes.
5. Flip the ravioli after 8 minutes and resume cooking. Serve warm.

Nutrition:
Calories: 124 Cal
Protein: 4.5 g
Carbs: 27.5 g
Fat: 3.5 g

220.Eggplant Fries

Preparation Time: 10 minutes
Cooking Time: 20 minutes
Servings: 4
Ingredients:

- 1/2 cup panko breadcrumbs
- 1/2 tsp. salt
- 1 eggplant, peeled and sliced
- 1 cup egg, whisked

Directions:

1.Toss the breadcrumbs with salt in a tray.
2.Dip the eggplant in the whisked egg and coat with the crumb's mixture.
3.Place the eggplant slices in the Air Fryer basket. Put the basket inside the Air Fryer toaster oven and close the lid.
4. Select the Air Fry mode at 400°F temperature for 20 minutes.
5.Flip the slices after 10 minutes, then resume cooking. Serve warm.

Nutrition:
Calories: 110 Cal
Protein: 5 g
Carbs: 12.8 g
Fat: 11.9 g

221.Stuffed Eggplants

Preparation Time: 10 minutes
Cooking Time: 38 minutes
Servings: 4
Ingredients:

- eggplants, cut in half lengthwise
- 1/2 cup shredded cheddar cheese
- 1/2 can (7.5 oz.) chili without beans
- 1 tsp. kosher salt

FOR SERVING

- 1 tbsp. cooked bacon bits
- 1 tbsp. sour cream
- Fresh scallions, thinly sliced

Directions:

1.Place the eggplants halves in the Air Fryer toaster oven and close the lid.
2.Select the Air Fry mode at 390°F temperature for 35 minutes.
3.Top each eggplant half with chili, cheese, and salt.
4.Place the halves in a baking pan and return to the oven. Select the Broil mode at 375°F temperature for 3 minutes.
5. Garnish with bacon bits, sour cream, and scallions. Serve.

Nutrition:

Calories: 113 Cal
Protein: 9.2 g
Carbs: 13 g
Fat: 21 g

222.Bacon Poppers

Preparation Time: 10 minutes
Cooking Time: 15 minutes
Servings: 4
Ingredients:

- strips bacon, crispy cooked

Dough:

- 2/3 cup water
- tbsp. butter
- 1 tbsp. bacon fat
- 1 tsp. kosher salt
- 2/3 cup all-purpose flour
- eggs
- oz. Cheddar cheese, shredded
- ½ cup jalapeno peppers
- A pinch pepper
- A pinch black pepper

Directions:

1.Whisk butter with water and salt in a skillet over medium heat. Stir in flour, then stir cook for about 3 minutes.
2.Transfer this flour to a bowl, then whisk in eggs and the rest of the ingredients.
3.Fold in bacon and mix well. Wrap this dough in a plastic sheet and refrigerate for 30 minutes. Make small balls out of this dough.
4.Place these bacon balls in the Air Fryer toaster oven and close the lid.
5.Select the Air Fry mode at 390°F temperature for 15 minutes. Flip the balls after 7 minutes, then resume cooking. Serve warm.

Nutrition:

Calories: 240 Cal
Protein: 14.9 g
Carbs: 7.1 g
Fat: 22.5 g

223.Stuffed Jalapeno

Preparation Time: 10 minutes
Cooking Time: 10 minutes
Servings: 4
Ingredients:

- 1 lb. ground pork sausage
- 1 (8 oz.) package cream cheese, softened
- 1 cup shredded Parmesan cheese
- 1 lb. large fresh jalapeno peppers halved lengthwise and seeded
- 1 (8 oz.) bottle Ranch dressing

Directions:

1.Mix pork sausage ground with ranch dressing and cream cheese in a bowl.
2.But the jalapeno in half and remove their seeds.
3.Divide the cream cheese mixture into the jalapeno halves. Place the jalapeno pepper in a baking tray.
4.Set the Baking tray inside the Air Fryer toaster oven and close the lid.
5.Select the Bake mode at 350°F temperature for 10 minutes. Serve warm.

Nutrition:

Calories: 168 Cal
Protein: 9.4 g
Carbs: 12.1 g
Fat: 21.2 g

224.Creamy Mushrooms

Preparation Time: 10 minutes
Cooking Time: 15 minutes
Servings: 24
Ingredients:

- 20 mushrooms

- 1 orange bell pepper, diced
- 1 onion, diced
- slices bacon, diced
- 1 cup shredded Cheddar cheese
- 1 cup sour cream

Directions:

1.First, sauté the mushroom stems with onion, bacon, and bell pepper in a pan.
2.After 5 minutes of cooking, add 1 cup cheese and sour cream. Cook for 2 minutes.
3.Place the mushroom caps on the Air Fryer basket crisper plate.
4.Stuff each mushroom with the cheese-vegetable mixture and top them with cheddar cheese.
5.Insert the basket back insider and select Air Fry mode for 8 minutes at 350°F.
6.Serve warm.

Nutrition:

Calories: 101 Cal
Protein: 8.8 g
Carbs: 25 g
Fat: 12.2 g

225.Italian Corn Fritters

Preparation Time: 10 minutes
Cooking Time: 3 minutes
Servings: 4
Ingredients:

- 2 cups frozen corn kernels
- 1/3 cup finely ground cornmeal
- 1/3 cup flour
- ½ tsp. salt
- ¼ tsp. pepper
- ½ tsp. baking powder
- Onion powder, to taste
- Garlic powder, to taste
- ¼ tsp. paprika
- 1 tbsp. green chilies with juices
- 1 tbsp. almond milk
- ¼ cup chopped Italian parsley

Directions:

1.Beat cornmeal with flour, baking powder, parsley, seasonings in a bowl. Blend 3 tbsp. almond milk with 1 cup corn, black pepper, and salt in a food processor until smooth.
2.Stir in the flour mixture, then mix until smooth. Spread this corn mixture on a baking tray lined with wax paper.
3.Set the baking tray inside the Air Fryer toaster oven and close the lid.
4.Select the bake mode at 350°F temperature for 2 minutes. Slice and serve.

Nutrition:

Calories: 146 Cal
Protein: 6.3 g
Carbs: 18.8 g
Fat: 4.5 g

226.Artichoke Fries

Preparation Time: 8 minutes
Cooking Time: 13 minutes
Servings: 6
Ingredients:

- 1 oz. can artichoke hearts
- 1 cup flour
- 1 cup almond milk
- ½ tsp. garlic powder
- ¾ tsp. salt
- ¼ tsp. black pepper, or to taste

For Dry Mix:

- 1 ½ cup panko breadcrumbs
- ½ tsp. paprika
- ¼ tsp. salt

Directions:

1.Whisk the wet ingredients in a bowl until smooth, and mix the dry ingredients in a separate bowl.
2.First, dip the artichokes quarters in the wet mixture, then coat with the dry panko mixture.
3.Place the artichokes hearts in the Air Fryer basket. Insert the basket inside the Air Fryer toaster oven and close the lid.
4. Select the Air Fry mode at 340°F temperature for 13 minutes. Serve warm.

Nutrition:

Calories: 199 Cal
Protein: 9.4 g
Carbs: 15.9 g
Fat: 4 g

227.Crumbly Beef Meatballs

Preparation Time: 8 minutes
Cooking Time: 20 minutes
Servings: 6
Ingredients:

- lbs. of ground beef
- 4 large eggs
- 1-1/4 cup panko breadcrumbs
- 1/4 cup chopped fresh parsley
- 1 tsp. dried oregano

- 1/4 cup grated Parmigianino Reggiano
- 1 small clove garlic chopped
- salt and pepper to taste
- 1 tsp. vegetable oil

Directions:

1.Thoroughly mix beef with eggs, crumbs, parsley, and the rest of the ingredients.
2.Make small meatballs out of this mixture and place them in the basket.
3.Place the basket inside the Air Fryer toaster oven and close the lid.
4.Select the Air Fry mode at 350°F temperature for 13 minutes.
5.Toss the meatballs after 5 minutes and resume cooking.
6.Serve fresh.

Nutrition:
Calories: 221 Cal
Protein: 25.1 g
Carbs: 11.2 g
Fat: 16.5 g

228.Pork Stuffed Dumplings

Preparation Time: 15 minutes
Cooking Time: 12 minutes
Servings: 3
Ingredients:

- 1 tsp. canola oil
- 2 cups chopped book Choy
- 1 tbsp. chopped fresh ginger
- 1 tbsp. chopped garlic
- oz. ground pork
- 1/4 tsp. crushed red pepper
- 18 dumpling wrappers
- Cooking spray
- tbsp. rice vinegar
- tsp. lower-sodium soy sauce
- 1 tsp. toasted sesame oil
- 1/2 tsp. packed light Sugar
- 1 tbsp. finely chopped scallions

Directions:

1.In a greased skillet, sauté bok choy for 8 minutes, then add ginger and garlic. Cook for 1 minute.
2.Transfer the bok choy to a plate.
3.Add pork and red pepper, then mix well. Place the dumpling wraps on the working surface and divide the pork fillings on the dumpling wraps.
4.Wet the edges of the wraps and pinch them together to seal the filling.
5.Place the dumpling in the Air Fryer basket.
6.Set the Air Fryer basket inside the Air Fryer toaster oven and close the lid.
7.Select the Air Fry mode at 375°F temperature for 12 minutes.
8. Flip the dumplings after 6 minutes, then resume cooking.
9.Serve fresh.

Nutrition:
Calories: 172 Cal
Protein: 2.1 g
Carbs: 18.6 g
Fat: 10.7 g

229.Panko Tofu with Mayo Sauce

Preparation Time: 10 minutes
Cooking Time: 20 minutes
Servings: 4
Ingredients:

- tofu cutlets

For the Marinade

- 1 tbsp toasted sesame oil
- 1/4 cup soy sauce
- 1 tsp rice vinegar
- 1/2 tsp garlic powder
- 1 tsp. ground ginger

Make the Tofu:

- 1/2 cup vegan mayo
- 1 cup panko breadcrumbs
- 1 tsp. of sea salt

Directions:

1.Whisk the marinade ingredients in a bowl and add tofu cutlets. Mix well to coat the cutlets.
2.Cover and marinate for 1 hour. Meanwhile, whisk crumbs with salt and mayo in a bowl.
3.Coat the cutlets with crumbs mixture. Place the tofu cutlets in the Air Fryer basket.
4.Select the Air Fry mode at 370°F temperature for 20 minutes. Flip the cutlets after 10 minutes, then resume cooking.
5.Serve warm.

Nutrition:
Calories: 151 Cal
Protein: 1.9 g
Carbs: 6.9 g
Fat: 8.6 g

230.Garlicky Bok Choy

Preparation Time: 10 minutes
Cooking Time: 10 minutes
Servings: 2
Ingredients:

- bunches baby book Choy
- Spray oil
- 1 tsp. garlic powder

Directions:
1.Toss bok choy with garlic powder and spread them in the Air Fryer basket.
2.Spray them with cooking oil.
3.Place the basket inside the Air Fryer toaster oven and close the lid.
4.Select the Air Fry mode at 350°F temperature for 6 minutes. Serve fresh.
Nutrition:
Calories: 81 Cal
Protein: 0.4 g
Carbs: 4.7 g
Fat: 8.3 g

231.Seasoned Cauliflower Chunks

Preparation Time: 10 minutes
Cooking Time: 15 minutes
Servings: 4
Ingredients:

- 1 cauliflower head, diced into chunks
- ½ cup unsweetened milk
- 1 tbsp. mayo
- ¼ cup all-purpose flour
- ¾ cup almond meal
- ¼ cup almond meal
- 1 tsp. onion powder
- 1 tsp. garlic powder
- 1 tsp. of sea salt
- ½ tsp. paprika
- Pinch of black pepper
- Cooking oil spray

Directions:
1.Toss cauliflower with the rest of the ingredients in a bowl, then transfers to the Air Fryer basket.
2.Spray them with cooking oil.
3. Set the basket inside the Air Fryer toaster oven and close the lid.
4.Select the Air Fry mode at 400°F temperature for 15 minutes.
5.Toss well and serve warm.
Nutrition:
Calories: 137 Cal
Protein: 6.1 g
Carbs: 26 g
Fat: 8 g

Chapter 22.Desserts

232.Mini Cheesecakes

Preparation Time: 15 minutes
Cooking Time: 10 minutes
Servings: 2
Ingredients:

- ¾ cup erythritol
- 4 eggs
- 1 teaspoon vanilla extract
- ½ teaspoon fresh lemon juice
- oz. Cream cheese, softened
- tablespoon sour cream

Directions:

1.In a blender, add the erythritol, eggs, vanilla extract, and lemon juice and pulse until smooth.
2.Add the cream cheese and sour cream and pulse until smooth.
3.Place the mixture into 2 (4-inch) springform pans evenly.
4.Press the "power button" of the air fry oven and turn the dial to select the "air fry" mode.
5.Press the time button and again turn the dial to set the cooking time to 10 minutes.
6.Now push the temp button and rotate the dial to set the temperature at 350 degrees f.
7.Press the "start/pause" button to start.
8.When the unit beeps to show that it is preheated, open the lid.
9.Arrange the pans in the "air fry basket" and insert in the oven.
10. Place the pans onto a wire rack to cool completely.
11. Refrigerate overnight before serving.

Nutrition:

Calories 886
Total fat 86 g
Saturated fat 52.8 g
Cholesterol 418 mg
Sodium 740 mg
Total carbs 7.2 g
Fiber 0 g
Sugar 1.1 g
Protein 23.1 g

233.Vanilla Cheesecake

Preparation Time: 15 minutes
Cooking Time: 14 minutes
Servings: 6
Ingredients:

- 1 cup honey graham cracker crumbs
- 3 tablespoons unsalted butter, softened
- 1 (453.592g). Cream cheese, softened
- ½ cup sugar
- 2 large eggs
- ½ teaspoon vanilla extract

Directions:

1.Line a round baking pan with parchment paper.
2.For crust: in a bowl, add the graham cracker crumbs, and butter.
3.Place the crust into baking dish and press to smooth.
4.Press "power button" of air fry oven and turn the dial to select the "air fry" mode.
5.Press the time button and again turn the dial to set the cooking time to 4 minutes.
6.Now push the temp button and rotate the dial to set the temperature at 350 degrees f.
7.Press "start/pause" button to start.
8.When the unit beeps to show that it is preheated, open the lid.
9.Arrange the baking pan of crust in "air fry basket" and insert in the oven.
10. Place the crust aside to cool for about 10 minutes.
11. Meanwhile, in a bowl, add the cream cheese, and sugar and whisk until smooth.
12. Now, place the eggs, one at a time and whisk until mixture becomes creamy.
13. Add the vanilla extract and mix well.
14. Place the cream cheese mixture evenly over the crust.
15. Press "power button" of air fry oven and turn the dial to select the "air fry" mode.
16. Press the time button and again turn the dial to set the cooking time to 10 minutes.
17. Now push the temp button and rotate the dial to set the temperature at 350 degrees f.
18. Press "start/pause" button to start.
19. When the unit beeps to show that it is preheated, open the lid.
20. Arrange the baking pan of crust in "air fry basket" and insert in the oven.
21. Place the pan onto a wire rack to cool completely.

22. Refrigerate overnight before serving.

Nutrition:

Calories 470
Total fat 33.9 g
Saturated fat 20.6 g
Cholesterol 155 mg
Sodium 42 mg
Total carbs 34.9 g
Fiber 0.5 g
Sugar 22 g
Protein 9.4 g

234.Ricotta Cheesecake

Preparation Time: 15 minutes
Cooking Time: 25 minutes
Servings: 8
Ingredients:

- 17.6 oz. Ricotta cheese
- 4 eggs
- ¾ cup sugar
- 2 tablespoons corn starch
- 1 tablespoon fresh lemon juice
- 2 teaspoons vanilla extract
- 1 teaspoon fresh lemon zest, finely grated

Directions:

1.In a large bowl, place all ingredients and mix until well combined.
2.Place the mixture into a baking pan.
3.Press the "power button" of the air fry oven and turn the dial to select the "air fry" mode.
4.Press the time button and again turn the dial to set the cooking time to 25 minutes.
5.Now push the temp button and rotate the dial to set the temperature at 320 degrees f.
6.Press the "start/pause" button to start.
7.When the unit beeps to show that it is preheated, open the lid.
8.Arrange the pan in the "air fry basket" and insert in the oven.
9.Place the cake pan onto a wire rack to cool completely.
10. Refrigerate overnight before serving.

Nutrition:

Calories 197
Total fat 6.6 g
Saturated fat 3.6 g
Cholesterol 81 mg
Sodium 102 mg
Total carbs 25.7 g
Fiber 0 g
Sugar 19.3 g
Protein 9.2 g

235.Pecan Pie

Preparation Time: 15 minutes
Cooking Time: 35 minutes
Servings: 5
Ingredients:

- ¾ cup brown sugar
- ¼ cup caster sugar
- 1/3 cup butter, melted
- 4 large eggs
- 1¾ tablespoons flour
- 1 tablespoon milk
- 1 teaspoon vanilla extract
- 1 cup pecan halves
- 1 frozen pie crust, thawed

Directions:

1.In a large bowl, mix together the sugars and butter.
2.Add the eggs and whisk until foamy.
3.Add the flour, milk, and vanilla extract and whisk until well combined.
4.Fold in the pecan halves.
5.Grease a pie pan.
6.Arrange the crust on the bottom of the prepared pie pan.
7.Place the pecan mixture over the crust evenly.
8.Press the "power button" of the air fry oven and turn the dial to select the "air fry" mode.
9.Press the time button and again turn the dial to set the cooking time to 22 minutes.
10. Now push the temp button and rotate the dial to set the temperature at 300 degrees f.
11. Press the "start/pause" button to start.
12. When the unit beeps to show that it is preheated, open the lid.
13. Arrange the pan in the "air fry basket" and insert in the oven.
14. After 22 minutes of cooking, to set the temperature at w85 degrees f for 13 minutes.
15. Place the pie pan onto a wire rack to cool for about 10-15 minutes before serving.

Nutrition:

Calories 501
Total fat 35 g
Saturated fat 10.8 g
Cholesterol 107 mg
Sodium 187 mg
Total carbs 44.7 g

Fiber 2.9 g
Sugar 36.7 g
Protein 6.2 g

236.Fruity Crumble

Preparation Time: 15 minutes
Cooking Time: 20 minutes
Servings: 4
Ingredients:

- ½ lb. (226.8g) Fresh apricots, pitted and cubed
- 1 cup fresh blackberries
- 1/3 cup sugar, divided
- 1 tablespoon fresh lemon juice
- 7/8 cup flour
- Pinch of salt
- 1 tablespoon cold water
- ¼ cup chilled butter, cubed

Directions:

1.Grease a baking pan.
2.In a large bowl, mix well apricots, blackberries, 2 tablespoons of sugar, and lemon juice.
3.Spread apricot mixture into the prepared baking pan.
4.In another bowl, add the flour, remaining sugar, salt, water, and butter and mix until a crumbly mixture form.
5.Spread the flour mixture over the apricot mixture evenly.
6.Press the "power button" of the air fry oven and turn the dial to select the "air fry" mode.
7.Press the time button and again turn the dial to set the cooking time to 20 minutes.
8.Now push the temp button and rotate the dial to set the temperature at 390 degrees f.
9.Press the "start/pause" button to start.
10. When the unit beeps to show that it is preheated, open the lid.
11. Arrange the pan in the "air fry basket" and insert in the oven.
12. Place the pan onto a wire rack to cool for about 10-15 minutes before serving.

Nutrition:

Calories 307
Total fat 12.4 g
Saturated fat 7.4 g
Cholesterol 31 mg
Sodium 123 mg
Total carbs 47.3 g
Fiber 3.8 g
Sugar 23.7 g
Protein 4.2 g

237.Cherry Clafoutis

Preparation Time: 15 minutes
Cooking Time: 25 minutes
Servings: 4
Ingredients:

- 1½ cups fresh cherries, pitted
- 2 tablespoons vodka
- ¼ cup flour
- 2 tablespoons sugar
- Pinch of salt
- ½ cup sour cream
- 1 egg
- 1 tablespoon butter
- ¼ cup powdered sugar

Directions:

1.In a bowl, mix together the cherries and vodka.
2.In another bowl, mix together the flour, sugar, and salt.
3.Add the sour cream and egg and mix until a smooth dough form.
4.Grease a cake pan.
5.Place flour mixture evenly into the prepared cake pan.
6.Spread cherry mixture over the dough.
7.Place butter on top in the form of dots.
8.Press the "power button" of the air fry oven and turn the dial to select the "air fry" mode.
9.Press the time button and again turn the dial to set the cooking time to 25 minutes.
10. Now push the temp button and rotate the dial to set the temperature at 355 degrees f.
11. Press the "start/pause" button to start.
12. When the unit beeps to show that it is preheated, open the lid.
13. Arrange the pan in the "air fry basket" and insert in the oven.
14. Place the pan onto a wire rack to cool for about 10-15 minutes before serving.
15. Now, invert the clafoutis onto a platter and sprinkle with powdered sugar.
16. Cut the clafoutis into desired size slices and serve warm.

Nutrition:

Calories 241
Total fat 10.1 g
Saturated fat 5.9 g
Cholesterol 61 mg

Sodium 90 mg
Total carbs 29 g
Fiber 1.3 g
Sugar 20.6 g
Protein 3.9 g

238.Apple Bread Pudding

Preparation Time: 15 minutes
Cooking Time: 44 minutes
Servings: 8
Ingredients:
For bread pudding:

- 10½ oz. Bread, cubed
- ½ cup apple, peeled, cored and chopped
- ½ cup raisins
- ¼ cup walnuts, chopped
- 1½ cups milk
- ¾ cup water
- 2 tablespoons honey
- 2 teaspoons ground cinnamon
- 2 teaspoons cornstarch
- 1 teaspoon vanilla extract

For topping:

- 1 1/3 cups plain flour
- 3/5 cup brown sugar
- tablespoons butter

Directions:
1.In a large bowl, mix together the bread, apple, raisins, and walnuts.
2.In another bowl, add the remaining pudding ingredients and mix until well combined.
3.Add the milk mixture into the bread mixture and mix until well combined.
4.Refrigerate for about 15 minutes, tossing occasionally.
5.For topping: in a bowl, mix together the flour and sugar.
6.With a pastry cutter, cut in the butter until a crumbly mixture form.
7.Place the mixture into 2 baking pans and spread the topping mixture on top of each.
8.Press the "power button" of the air fry oven and turn the dial to select the "air fry" mode.
9.Press the time button and again turn the dial to set the cooking time to 22 minutes.
10. Now push the temp button and rotate the dial and set the temperature at 355 degrees f.
11. Press the "start/pause" button to start.
12. When the unit beeps to show that it is preheated, open the lid.
13. Arrange 1 pan in "air fry basket" and insert in the oven.
14. Place the pan onto a wire rack to cool slightly before serving.
15. Repeat with the remaining pan.
16. Serve warm.

Nutrition:
Calories 432
Total fat 14.8 g
Saturated fat 7.4 g
Cholesterol 30 mg
Sodium 353mg
Total carbs 69.1 g
Fiber 2.8 g
Sugar 32 g
Protein 7.9 g

239.Masala Cashew

Preparation Time: 25 minutes
Cooking Time: 50 Minutes
Servings: 2
Ingredients

- oz Greek yogurt
- 1 tbsp mango powder
- 8¾ oz cashew nuts
- Salt and pepper to taste
- 1 tsp coriander powder
- ½ tsp masala powder
- ½ tsp black pepper powder

Directions
1.Preheat your Fryer to 240 F.
2. In a bowl, mix all powders. Season with salt and pepper.
3. Add cashews and toss to coat well.
4. Place the cashews in your air fryer's basket and cook for 15 minutes. Serve with a garnish of basil.

Nutrition:
Calories: 202;
Fat: 6;
Fiber: 3;
Carbs: 17;
Protein: 10

Chapter 23.Dessert 2

240.Donuts Pudding

Preparation Time: 15 minutes
Cooking Time: 1 hour
Servings: 6
Ingredients:

- glazed donuts, cut into small pieces
- ¾ cup frozen sweet cherries
- ½ cup raisins
- ½ cup semi-sweet chocolate baking chips.
- ¼ cup sugar
- 1 teaspoon ground cinnamon
- 4 egg yolks
- 1½ cups whipping cream

Directions:

1.In a large bowl, mix together the donut pieces, cherries, raisins, chocolate chips, sugar, and cinnamon.
2.In another bowl, add the egg yolks and whipping cream and whisk until well combined.
3.Add the egg yolk mixture into the doughnut mixture and mix well.
4.Line a baking dish with a piece of foil.
5.Place donuts mixture into the prepared baking pan.
6.Press the "power button" of the air fry oven and turn the dial to select the "air fry" mode.
7.Press the time button and again turn the dial to set the cooking time to 60 minutes.
8.Now push the temp button and rotate the dial to set the temperature at 360 degrees f.
9.Press the "start/pause" button to start.
10. When the unit beeps to show that it is preheated, open the lid.
11. Arrange the pan in the "air fry basket" and insert it in the oven.
12. Place the pan onto a wire rack to cool for about 10-15 minutes before serving.
13. Serve warm.

Nutrition:
Calories 537
Total fat 28.7 g
Saturated fat 12.2 g
Cholesterol 173 mg
Sodium 194 mg
Total carbs 65.1 g
Fiber 2.3 g
Sugar 32.8 g
Protein 6.5 g

241.Buttery Scallops

Preparation Time: 10 minutes
Cooking Time: 25 minutes
Servings: 8
Ingredients

- lb. (907.185g) Scallops
- 2 tablespoons butter, melted
- 2 tablespoons dry white wine
- 1 tablespoon lemon juice
- 1/2 cup parmesan cheese, grated
- 1 teaspoon salt
- 1/2 teaspoon black pepper
- 1 teaspoon garlic powder
- 1 teaspoon dried parsley
- 1/8 teaspoon cayenne pepper
- 1/4 teaspoon sweet paprika
- 2 tablespoons parsley chopped

Directions:

1.Mix everything in a bowl except scallops.
2.Toss in scallops and mix well to coat them.
3.Spread the scallops with the sauce on a baking tray.
4.Press the "power button" of the air fry oven and turn the dial to select the "bake" mode.
5.Press the time button and again turn the dial to set the cooking time to 25 minutes.
6.Now push the temp button and rotate the dial to set the temperature at 350 degrees f.
7.Once preheated, place the scallop's baking tray in the oven and close its lid.
8.Serve warm.

Nutrition:
Calories 227
Total fat 10.1g
Saturated fat 5.7g
Cholesterol 89mg
Sodium 388mg
Total carbohydrate 5.6g
Dietary fiber 0.1g
Total sugars 0.2g
Protein 27.8g

242.Crusted Scallops

Preparation Time: 10 minutes
Cooking Time: 20 minutes
Servings: 4

Ingredients

- 1 1/2 lbs. (680.389g) Bay scallops, rinsed
- garlic cloves, minced
- 1/2 cup panko crumbs
- 1 teaspoon onion powder
- 2 tablespoons butter, melted
- 1/2 teaspoon cayenne pepper
- 1 teaspoon garlic powder
- 1/4 cup parmesan cheese, shredded

Directions:

1.Mix everything in a bowl except scallops.
2.Toss in scallops and mix well to coat them.
3.Spread the scallops with the sauce in a baking tray.
4.Press the "power button" of the air fry oven and turn the dial to select the "bake" mode.
5.Press the time button and again turn the dial to set the cooking time to 20 minutes.
6.Now push the temp button and rotate the dial to set the temperature at 400 degrees f.
7.Once preheated, place the scallop's baking tray in the oven and close its lid.

Nutrition:

Calories 242
Total fat 11.1g
Saturated fat 6.4g
Cholesterol 65mg
Sodium 500mg
Total carbohydrate 11.1g
Dietary fiber 0.7g
Total sugars 0.9g
Protein 23.8g

243.Lobster Tails with White Wine Sauce

Preparation Time: 10 minutes
Cooking Time: 14 minutes
Servings: 4
Ingredients

- lobster tails, shell cut from the top
- 1/2 onion, quartered
- 1/2 cup butter
- 1/3 cup wine
- 1/4 cup honey
- garlic cloves crushed
- 1 tablespoon lemon juice
- 1 teaspoon salt or to taste
- Cracked pepper to taste
- Lemon slices to serve
- tablespoons fresh chopped parsley

Directions:

1.Place the lobster tails in the oven's baking tray.
2.Whisk the rest of the ingredients in a bowl and pour over the lobster tails.
3.Press the "power button" of the air fry oven and turn the dial to select the "broil" mode.
4.Press the time button and again turn the dial to set the cooking time to 14 minutes.
5.Now push the temp button and rotate the dial to set the temperature at 350 degrees f.
6.Once preheated, place the lobster's baking tray in the oven and close its lid.
7.Serve warm.

Nutrition:

Calories 340
Total fat 23.1g
Saturated fat 14.6g
Cholesterol 61mg
Sodium 1249mg
Total carbohydrate 20.4g
Dietary fiber 0.3g
Total sugars 18.1g
Protein 0.7g

244.Broiled Lobster Tails

Preparation Time: 10 minutes
Cooking Time: 6 minutes
Servings: 4
Ingredients

- lobster tails, shell cut from the top
- 1/2 cup butter, melted
- 1/2 teaspoon ground paprika
- Salt to taste
- White pepper, to taste
- 1 lemon, juiced

Directions:

1.Place the lobster tails in the oven's baking tray.
2.Whisk the rest of the ingredients in a bowl and pour over the lobster tails.
3.Press the "power button" of the air fry oven and turn the dial to select the "broil" mode.
4.Press the time button and again turn the dial to set the cooking time to 6 minutes.
5.Now push the temp button and rotate the dial to set the temperature at 350 degrees f.

6.Once preheated, place the lobster's baking tray in the oven and close its lid.
7.Serve warm.

Nutrition:
Calories 227
Total fat 23.1g
Saturated fat 14.6g
Cholesterol 61mg
Sodium 414mg
Total carbohydrate 0.2g
Dietary fiber 0.1g
Total sugars 0.1g
Protein 20.3g

245.Paprika Lobster Tail

Preparation Time: 10 minutes
Cooking Time: 10 minutes
Servings: 4
Ingredients

- (4 to 6 oz) lobster tails, shell cut from the top
- 1/8 teaspoon salt
- 1/8 teaspoon black pepper
- 1/8 teaspoon paprika
- 1 tablespoon butter
- 1/2 lemon, cut into wedges
- Chopped parsley for garnish

Directions:
1.Place the lobster tails in the oven's baking tray.
2.Whisk the rest of the ingredients in a bowl and pour over the lobster tails.
3.Press the "power button" of the air fry oven and turn the dial to select the "broil" mode.
4.Press the time button and again turn the dial to set the cooking time to 10 minutes.
5.Now push the temp button and rotate the dial to set the temperature at 350 degrees f.
6.Once preheated, place the lobster's baking tray in the oven and close its lid.
7.Serve warm.

Nutrition:
Calories 204
Total fat 12.5g
Saturated fat 7.5g
Cholesterol 196mg
Sodium 780mg
Total carbohydrate 0.2g
Dietary fiber 0.1g
Total sugars 0g
Protein 21.7g

246.Lobster Tails with Lemon Butter

Preparation Time: 10 minutes
Cooking Time: 8 minutes
Servings: 4
Ingredients

- lobster tails, shell cut from the top
- 1 tablespoon fresh parsley, chopped
- garlic cloves, pressed
- 1 teaspoon dijon mustard
- 1/4 teaspoon salt
- 1/8 teaspoon black pepper
- 1 1/2 tablespoon olive oil
- 1 1/2 tablespoon fresh lemon juice
- 1 tablespoon butter, divided

Directions:
1.Place the lobster tails in the oven's baking tray.
2.Whisk the rest of the ingredients in a bowl and pour over the lobster tails.
3.Press the "power button" of the air fry oven and turn the dial to select the "broil" mode.
4.Press the time button and again turn the dial to set the cooking time to 8 minutes.
5.Now push the temp button and rotate the dial to set the temperature at 350 degrees f.
6.Once preheated, place the lobster's baking tray in the oven and close its lid.
7.Serve warm.

Nutrition:
Calories 281
Total fat 18.1g
Saturated fat 8.4g
Cholesterol 242mg
Sodium 950mg
Total carbohydrate 0.8g
Dietary fiber 0.1g
Total sugars 0.2g
Protein 27.9g

247.Sheet Pan Seafood Bake

Preparation Time: 10 minutes
Cooking Time: 14 minutes
Servings: 4
Ingredients

- corn ears, husked and diced
- 1 lb. (453.592g) Red potatoes, boiled, diced

- lbs. (907.185g) Clams, scrubbed
- 1 lb. (453.592g) Shrimp, peeled and de-veined
- oz. Sausage, sliced
- 1/2 red onion, sliced
- lobster tails, peeled
- Black pepper to taste
- 1 lemon, cut into wedges
- 1 cup butter
- 2 teaspoons minced garlic
- 1 tablespoon old bay seasoning
- Fresh parsley for garnish

Directions:

1.Toss all the veggies, corn, seafood, oil, and seasoning in a baking tray.
2.Press the "power button" of the air fry oven and turn the dial to select the "broil" mode.
3.Press the time button and again turn the dial to set the cooking time to 14 minutes.
4.Now push the temp button and rotate the dial to set the temperature at 425 degrees f.
5.Once preheated, place the seafood's baking tray in the oven and close its lid.
6.Serve warm.

Nutrition:

Calories 532
Total fat 35.6g
Saturated fat 18.8g
Cholesterol 219mg
Sodium 1379mg
Total carbohydrate 26.3g
Dietary fiber 2.5g
Total sugars 4.4
Protein 28.7g

248.Orange Sponge Cake

Preparation Time: 50 minutes
Cooking Time: 14 minutes
Servings: 6
Ingredients

- oz sugar
- oz self-rising flour
- oz butter
- eggs
- 1 tsp baking powder
- 1 tsp vanilla extract
- Zest of 1 orange

Frosting:

- egg whites
- Juice of 1 orange
- 1 tsp orange food coloring
- Zest of 1 orange
- oz superfine sugar

Directions

1.Preheat Breville on bake function to 160 f and place all cake ingredients in a bowl and beat with an electric mixer. Transfer half of the batter into a prepared cake pan; bake for 15 minutes. Repeat the process for the other half of the batter.
2.Meanwhile, prepare the frosting by beating all frosting ingredients together. Spread the frosting mixture on top of one cake. Top with the other cake.

Nutrition:

Calories: 828,
Protein:11.46 g,
Fat: 39.77g,
Carbs: 107.89g

249.Apricot Crumble with Blackberries

Preparation Time: 30 minutes
Servings: 4
Ingredients

- ½ cups fresh apricots, de-stoned and cubed
- 1 cup fresh blackberries
- ½ cup sugar
- 1 tbsp lemon juice
- 1 cup flour
- Salt as needed
- 1 tbsp butter

Directions

1.Add the apricot cubes to a bowl and mix with lemon juice, 2 tbsp sugar, and blackberries. Scoop the mixture into a greased dish and spread it evenly. In another bowl, mix flour and remaining sugar.
2.Add 1 tbsp of cold water and butter and keep mixing until you have a crumbly mixture. Preheat Breville on bake function to 390 f and place the fruit mixture in the basket. Top with crumb mixture and cook for 20 minutes.

Nutrition:

Calories: 546,
Protein: 7g,

Fat: 5.23g,
Carbs: 102.53g

250.Apple & Cinnamon Pie

Preparation Time: 30 minutes
Cooking Time: 14 minutes
Servings: 9
Ingredients

- apples, diced
- oz butter, melted
- oz sugar
- 1 oz brown sugar
- 1 tsp cinnamon
- 1 egg, beaten
- large puff pastry sheets
- ¼ tsp salt

Directions

1.Whisk white sugar, brown sugar, cinnamon, salt, and butter together. Place the apples in a baking dish and coat them with the mixture. Place the baking dish in the toaster oven, and cook for 10 minutes at 350 f on bake function.

2.Meanwhile, roll out the pastry on a floured flat surface, and cut each sheet into 6 equal pieces. Divide the apple filling between the pieces. Brush the edges of the pastry squares with the egg.

3.Fold them and seal the edges with a fork. Place on a lined baking sheet and cook in the fryer at 350 f for 8 minutes. Flip over, increase the temperature to 390 f, and cook for 2 more minutes.

Nutrition:
Calories: 140,
Protein: 1.28g,
Fat: 6.33g,
Carbs: 21.19g

CPSIA information can be obtained
at www.ICGtesting.com
Printed in the USA
LVHW060837270323
742607LV00005B/101